Fluid, Electrolyte, Metabolic and Respiratory Acid-Base Management

Fluid, Electrolyte, Metabolic and Respiratory Acid-Base Management

A Vimala MBBS MD DM (Nephrology) FRCP (Lond)
Professor of Nephrology
Dr SMCSI Medical College
Karakonam, Thiruvananthapuram
Consultant Nephrologist
Dr Govindan's Hospital
Thiruvananthapuram, Kerala, India
Formerly
Vice Principal
Medical College
Kottayam, Kerala, India
E-mail: vimala52@rediffmail.com

Foreword
MA Muthusethupathi

JAYPEE BROTHERS MEDICAL PUBLISHERS (P) LTD

New Delhi • London • Philadelphia • Panama

Jaypee Brothers Medical Publishers (P) Ltd

Headquarters
Jaypee Brothers Medical Publishers (P) Ltd
4838/24, Ansari Road, Daryaganj
New Delhi 110 002, India
Phone: +91-11-43574357
Fax: +91-11-43574314
Email: jaypee@jaypeebrothers.com

J.P. Medical Ltd
83 Victoria Street, London
SW1H 0HW (UK)
Phone: +44-2031708910
Fax: +44 (0) 20 3086180
Email: info@jpmedpub.com

Jaypee Medical Inc.
The Bourse
111 South Independence Mall East
Suite 835, Philadelphia, PA 19106, USA
Phone: +1 267-519-9789
Email: jpmed.us@gmail.com

Jaypee-Highlights Medical Publishers Inc
City of Knowledge, Bld. 237, Clayton
Panama City, Panama
Phone: +1 507-301-0496
Fax: +1 507-301-0499
Email: cservice@jphmedical.com

Jaypee Brothers Medical Publishers (P) Ltd
17/1-B Babar Road, Block-B, Shaymali
Mohammadpur, Dhaka-1207
Bangladesh
Mobile: +08801912003485
Email: jaypeedhaka@gmail.com

Jaypee Brothers Medical Publishers (P) Ltd
Bhotahity, Kathmandu
Nepal
Phone: +977-9741283608
Email: kathmandu@jaypeebrothers.com

Website: www.jaypeebrothers.com
Website: www.jaypeedigital.com

Fluid, Electrolyte, Metabolic and Respiratory Acid-Base Management

First Edition: **2014**

ISBN 978-93-5152-193-8

Printed at Rajkamal Electric Press, Plot No. 2, Phase-IV, Kundli, Haryana.

Dedicated to

My beloved parents
Sri P Padmanabha Iyer and
Smt Avadai Ammal
&
My esteemed teacher
Professor VC Mathew Roy

Contributors

A Vimala MBBS MD DM (Nephrology) FRCP (Lond)
Professor of Nephrology
Dr SMCSI Medical College
Karakonam, Thiruvananthapuram
Consultant Nephrologist
Dr Govindan's Hospital
Thiruvananthapuram, Kerala, India
Formerly
Vice Principal
Medical College
Kottayam, Kerala, India

G Krishnakumar MD (Gen Med) DA EDIC FRCP
Physician and Intensivist
Dr Govindan's Hospital
Thiruvananthapuram, Kerala, India

R Kasi Visweswaran MD DM FRCP
Professor and Head
Department of Nephrology
Pushpagiri Medical College
Thiruvalla
Senior Consultant Nephrologist
Ananthapuri Hospital
Thiruvananthapuram, Kerala, India

Foreword

Ever since Claude Bernard formulated the concept that maintenance of the constancy of the internal environment (milieu interior) is the 'condition of free life', the central importance of the kidneys as a regulator of body fluid volume and composition has become increasingly studied and appreciated. Nephrologists with significant help from the internists have logically become the experts in the field of Fluid, Electrolyte and Acid-Base Disorders.

Because of the mathematical and physicochemical equations and formulae involved in its understanding, many doctors have put off this field of medicine, which, by common consent, has been considered a 'difficult' topic to teach and more difficult to practice at the bedside.

In actual fact, however, most of these Fluid, Electrolyte and Acid-Base problems are fairly easy to understand if one starts with some basic principles of chemistry and physiology. Correct understanding and application of these principles in practice lead to gratifying results for our patients, many of whose lives can thus be saved.

I feel that this topic by itself is quite interesting and intellectually challenging. What more can one ask in the field of study — beneficial to many and fascinating in its complexity?

Professor A Vimala is one of the brightest, conscientious and hard-working teachers and practitioners of Nephrology in our country today. Her commitment and teaching skills are truly extraordinary. It is fortunate indeed that she has chosen to write a book on this exciting topic for the benefit of all the students and teachers of medicine.

This book begins by describing the principles of Fluid and Electrolyte Physiology and goes on to discuss the various disorders encountered in practice. Section 2 describes an approach to Acid-Base disorders, starting with physiological principles and goes on to discuss the various disorders in a simple and easy-to-understand manner. My friend and esteemed colleague Professor R Kasi Visweswaran has contributed the chapters on Potassium abnormality and Metabolic Alkalosis which bears his hallmark of erudition and clarity.

I must mention that the text is interspersed with practical, clinical examples which go a long way in making this book more interesting and lively.

A section on the interpretation of Arterial Blood Gas studies has been included so that the readers of the book can learn the logical practical approach to Acid-Base problems in actual clinical practice.

One chapter on the Stewart approach to acid-base makes the text up-to-date regarding some important new advances in this field. It is a commendable effort. Dr G Krishnakumar, a dedicated intensivist, has tried his level best to make this complex chapter simple. He also has made a succinct presentation on respiratory acidosis, alkalosis and ventilator management, which is a model of clarity.

I congratulate the author, Professor A Vimala for her praiseworthy effort in bringing a book, which should serve generations of medical students and young nephrologists. I hope it may also serve to attract more young physicians to this fascinating field of study.

This book is one of those really useful manuals which must be read, chewed, digested and assimilated, so that it can be easily and naturally applied in clinical practice to help a large number of patients.

May this book enjoy a great success that it so richly deserves!

Dr Professor MA Muthusethupathi
Formerly: Professor and Head, Department of Nephrology
Madras Medical College and Government General Hospital
Chennai, India

Preface

We medical professionals, like professionals in many other fields, are often circumscribed by our circumstances—gaps in research, exposure and the resultant understanding available at our disposal. In hindsight, we often wish we had the knowledge or the perspective at a specific point in time that could have helped us approach and resolve a case better. Of course, every generation of dedicated professionals tries to contribute its own bit by drawing on its own exposure to the latest in medical advancements and specific medical cases. We have tried to do our bit too through this book.

As doctors with years of medical experience, we have been fortunate enough to have got a closer look at a variety of cases and medical scenarios. These experiences, while shaping our own perspectives and knowledge, have also enabled us to understand the different approaches taken by the medical professionals to specific case management. They have also made us wonder at better alternatives. Three specific areas that we have observed closely have been fluid therapy, electrolyte and ventilator management in intensive care. These areas, while being an important aspect in the treatment of any condition, have also been throwing some unique challenges at us. Right from the basics of fluid electrolyte abnormalities, fluid therapy, and analysis of pulmonary physiology to the analysis of respiratory acid-base, interpretation of ABG, maintenance of H^+ ion balance and much more, there is often the need for a comprehensive approach. This book is an attempt to look at some such aforementioned situations and seeks to offer a better understanding and approach through specific case studies and examples.

We have drawn on a number of cases that we have personally come across and attended to and also on notes and observations gathered over the years of professional experience. We have also included details of the treatment given in each case. The idea is to offer some perspectives to young medical professionals so that they are better equipped to decide on the right approach to treatment, especially in the intensive care stage. So, we hope that postgraduate students, young medical professionals and others will benefit from our hindsight and take a judicious approach to handling intensive care patients.

A Vimala

Acknowledgments

A venture of this kind owes its origins to many factors, not the least of them being the people who shape our perspectives and push us towards greater goals. I would first like to thank Professor MA Muthusethupathi, Former Professor and Head, Department of Nephrology, Madras Medical College, Chennai, India for being there for me as a mentor and giving me the right professional inputs. The same may be said of Professor S Krishnakumar, Former Professor of Nephrology, Medical College, Thiruvananthapuram, India, whom I would like to thank for guiding me professionally.

I must also say that this book would have remained a mere dream had it not been for the help of a few people who ought to be mentioned here. From sowing the seeds of the idea to giving the right dose of inspiration and supporting through valuable suggestions and other help, there have been many people who were the driving force behind this book.

I express my sincere gratitude to Professor R Kasi Visweswaran and Dr G Krishnakumar for contributing important chapters to this text.

First, a big thanks to Professor K Lalitha, Consultant Gynecologist, SUT Hospital, Thiruvananthapuram, for being the motivation behind this book.

I would also like to thank Dr Godwin, Dr Murali and Dr Jigy Joseph, who were of invaluable help, without which this book would have been impossible. Also, a special thanks to all my dear students, the ones who keep my professional spirit alive. They were of great help during the course of writing this book.

An initiative of this kind needs a focused direction of energy and commitment, which is possible only with a strong family support. And I must say I have been fortunate in this regard. I would like to thank my brother and sisters, brothers-in-law, sister-in-law and my nieces and nephews—Shalini,

Vivek, Gowri, Sharanya, Ananth and Nandini, all of whom supported me immensely as I threw myself into this book. I acknowledge my patients for whom it is a privilege to care.

My sincere appreciation also goes to Shri Jitendar P Vij (Group Chairman), Mr Ankit Vij (Managing Director) and Mr Tarun Duneja (Director-Publishing) of M/s Jaypee Brothers Medical Publishers (P) Ltd, New Delhi, India for their support in this project.

Last, but not the least, I would like to thank the team at Jaypee Brothers Medical Publishers, New Delhi and at Kochi Branch for being instrumental in bringing out this book.

Contents

Section 1 — Fluid and Electrolyte Abnormalities

Section **1**

Fluid and Electrolyte Abnormalities

- Physiological principles, composition and distribution of parenteral fluids
- Fluid therapy in pathological states
- Sodium homeostasis and renal regulation of sodium
- Hyponatremia
- Hypernatremia
- Potassium — Renal and endocrine regulation
- Hypokalemia
- Hyperkalemia
- Calcium — Hypocalcemia and hypercalcemia

Physiological Principles, Composition and Distribution of Parenteral Fluids

A Vimala

Judicious and appropriate administration of fluids form an integral part in the management of both surgical and medical patients. A thorough understanding of the basic physiology and recognition of different pathological states will help in proper patient care. This will not only reduce morbidity and mortality but also prevent iatrogenic problems.

MILESTONES IN THE DEVELOPMENT OF FLUID THERAPY

- Dr Thomas Latta in May 15, 1832 used first therapeutic infusion of intravenous fluid.
- Dr William Brooke O'Shaughnessy in 1887 described "Milieu interior".
- Jacobus H. Vant Hoff described osmosis in 1887.
- James Blundell did first human to human blood transfusion for a lady who had postpartum hemorrhage.
- Karl Landsteiner in 1901 received Nobel prize for his discovery of blood groups.
- 1980s and 1990s saw the use of recombinant factors, blood substitutes and blood-conserving therapies.

MILESTONES IN THE DEVELOPMENT OF PARENTERAL SOLUTIONS

- The first synthetic colloid used in human beings was gelatin in 1915.

- James Gamble (United States), defined the extracellular fluid (ECF) and its response to loss in fasting.
  Gamble defined new terms like mEq/L to describe concentrations in solutions, and graphically related *cations and anions* via bar graphs, which are known as Gamblegrams in 1950.
- SAFE (saline versus albumin fluid evaluation) trial, relative safety of 4% albumin compared with 0.9% saline was studied in critically ill patients (2004).
- VISEP trial (volume substitution and insulin therapy in severe sepsis), evaluated adverse renal outcomes with hydroxyethyl starch administration in septic shock patients (2008).

Basic Physiology of Water Distribution

Total body water is distributed mainly between the intracellular fluid (ICF) and extracellular fluid (ECF). About 1 to 2% of body water is 'transcellular water' found in cerebrospinal fluid, the humors of the eye, digestive secretions, renal tubular fluid and urine. Transcellular fluids are separated from the ECF by an endothelium and a continuous epithelial layer.

In adults about 60% of the body weight consists of fluids. 60% of the total body water (i.e. 40% body weight) is intracellular and 40% is extracellular (i.e. 20% body weight). Of the extracellular fluid, 5% of the total body weight is in the intravascular compartment and 15% is in the interstitial compartment.

Total body water varies according to fat content, sex and age. Fat cells contain less water, so females and elderly individuals have less body water than adults. Infants have a body fluid content of 70–80%.

Distribution of water as % of body weight according to age and sex is shown in Table 1.1. Fluid volumes in various compartments for a 70 kg man is shown in Figure 1.1.

Table 1.1: Water as %age of body weight			
Build	*Infant*	*Male*	*Female*
Thin	70	65	55
Average	70	60	50
Fat	65	55	45

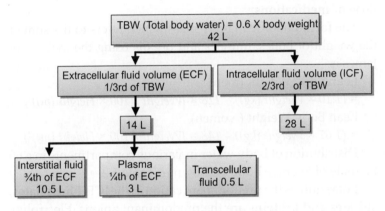

Fig. 1.1: Relationship between the volumes of major fluid compartments calculated for 70 kg man

Ideal body weight (IBW)

Ideal body weight can be used for nutritional assessment purposes. Can be calculated using Devine formula.

Ideal Body Weight (men)

= 50 + 2.3 kg [Height (in inches) – 60]

Ideal Body Weight (women)

= 45.5 + 2.3 kg [Height (in inches) – 60]

This formula is only an approximation, and is generally only applicable for people 60 inches (5 foot) tall or greater.

If the patient is severely underweight - (less than 80% of IBW) then use current weight for nutrient calculations.

If the patient is obese, use "adjusted body weight" for calculation.

Adjusted Body Weight = IBW + 0.25 (Usual Weight-IBW).

Examples: IBW for a lady of average build and height 65 inches is 45.5 + (5 × 2.3) = 57 kg

IBW for a man who is obese weight 80 kg and height 68 inches is 50 + (8 × 2.3) = 68.4 kg

Adjusted Body Weight = 68.4 + 0.25 (80 – 68.4) = 71.3 kg

Lean Body Weight is sometimes used for finding out the dose of medications.

The formula for lean body mass which refers to the sum of the weight of bones, muscles and organs using the method of James is:

Lean Body Weight (men)
= *(1.10 × Weight (kg)) – 128 × {Weight²/(100 × Height (m))²}*
Lean Body Weight (women)
= *(1.07 × Weight (kg)) – 148 × {Weight²/(100 × Height (m))²}*

Distribution of body water in various compartments in a 60 kg male of average build is shown in Table 1.2.

Potassium is the predominant cation in the ICF. **Phosphates, sulfates and proteins are** the predominant anions. Electrolyte composition of intracellular (ICF) is shown in Table 1.3.

Sodium is the predominant cation in ECF. **Chloride and bicarbonate** are the predominant anions. The composition of plasma and interstitial fluid is the same except for the protein content of plasma.

The distribution of cations and anions in plasma, plasma water, and interstitial fluid is shown in Tables 1.4 and 1.5 respectively.

Table 1.2: Distribution of water in 60 kg man

Compartment	Volume	In Liters
Total body fluid	60% of body weight	36 L
ICF	40% (2/3ʳᵈ) of body weight	24 L
ECF	20% (1/3ʳᵈ) of body weight	12 L
Interstitial fluid	3/4th of ECF	8 L
Plasma fluid	1/4th of ECF	4 L
Venous fluid	85% of plasma fluid	3.4 L
Arterial fluid	15% of plasma fluid	0.6 L

Table 1.3: ICF composition

Cations	mmol/L	Anions	mmol/L
K	150	PO_4 and SO_4	150
Mg	40	Protein	40
Na	10	HCO_3	10
Ca	0.001		
Total	200		200

Table 1.4 : ECF composition – Cations in mEq/L

Cations	Plasma	Plasma water	Interstitial fluid
Na	140	153	145
K	4	4.3	4
Ca	5	5.4	3
Mg	2	2.2	2
Total	151	165	154

Table 1.5: ECF composition – Anions mEq/L

Anions	Plasma	Plasma water	Interstitial fluid
Chloride	103	117	117
HCO_3	25	27	28
Protein	16	18	0
Others	7	9	9
Total	151	165	154

Concept of Third Space

The intravascular compartment is the first space and interstitium and cellular compartment form the second space. Third space is the space where the fluid does not collect in large volumes normally and the fluid accumulation is physiologically non-functional. Whenever, there is fluid loss into peritoneum, pericardial cavity, pleural cavity, lumen of the bowel, this is called third space loss. This is usually due to leakage of albumin into these areas. The identification and correction of third space loss is very important in correction of fluid deficit.

Electrolytes

- Sodium and potassium are important for maintaining osmolality and cell volume, generating the resting membrane potential and action potentials of excitable tissues.
- Calcium is largely an extracellular ion, but has an important role in the regulation of cell metabolism. In cardiac and skeletal muscle, calcium acts as the link between electrical activity and contraction. It also influences neuromuscular excitability and is required for blood clotting.
- Magnesium is mainly intracellular and is necessary for many intracellular enzyme systems, including oxidative phosphorylation and protein synthesis.
- *Chloride and bicarbonate* are the main extracellular anions. Chloride is important in the function of secretory and absorptive cells in the kidney and gastrointestinal tract.
- *Bicarbonate* is important in the control of pH and carbon dioxide transport.

The precise composition of the ICF is not identical across all cell types, and the ions are not distributed equally throughout the cell. In the RBC for example, the chloride ion concentration is relatively high (90 mmol/L) because of its role in carbon dioxide transport (chloride shift).

In muscle, calcium ions are sequestered in the sarcoplasmic reticulum where they have a fundamental role in excitation and contraction coupling.

Interstitial fluid is essentially an ultrafiltrate of plasma; the proteins remain in the circulation, which results in some differences in ionic concentrations - (Gibbs-Donnan equilibrium).

KEY POINT

Of the total body water around 2/3rd is in ICF and 1/3rd is in ECF. Only 1/12th of total body water is in the vascular compartment.

Basic fluid requirement is based on the fluid losses.

Table 1.6: Normal losses

Fluid	% of total loss	Volume in adult
Urine	60%	1440 mL (0.5–2 mL/kg/h)
Insensible loss (Skin and lungs)	35%	840 mL
Feces	5%	120 mL
Total		2400 mL

Fluid Losses

Loss is mainly as urine, through feces, insensible loss and sweat (Table 1.6).

Insensible Water Loss

This term refers to water loss due to:

- Transepidermal diffusion: Water that passes through the skin and is lost by evaporation.
- Evaporative water loss from the respiratory tract.

This cannot be measured and approximately estimated as 400 mL through skin and 400 mL through respiratory tract. The water loss through respiratory tract is variable: It is increased if minute ventilation increases and can be decreased if inspired gas is fully humidified at a temperature of 37°C (example: as in a ventilated ICU patient).

On an average day, activity increases the insensible respiratory water loss and the overall loss rises above minimum. The minimum insensible loss is around 50 *mL/h in unstressed hospitalized* patients. This solute-free water loss differs from sweating as sweat contains both water and solutes. Another difference is that sweat is produced in special glands in the skin.

50% of insensible loss is balanced by endogenous water production of around 400 mL.

Insensible loss is loss of pure water: There is no associated solute loss. In sweat, water and solutes are lost.

Based on the above facts normal maintenance fluid requirement is calculated as follows.

Fluid Requirement in Children

The total fluid requirement can be calculated according to"100/50/20" rule (Holliday–Segar method) (Table 1.7).

SCENARIO 1

A 12-year-old child, weighing 24 kg is to be given maintenance fluids. What will be his maintenance requirement? As shown in Table 1.7, total fluid required in 24 hours is 1580 mL and fluid requirement per hour is 64 mL (4/2/1 Rule-Table 1.8) Na required is $3 \times 16 = 48$ mmoles, K is around $2 \times 16 = 32$ mmoles (Table 1.10)

Based on this formula, total fluid required in 24 hours is $64 \times 24 = 1536$ mL

Approximate fluid requirement in adults is calculated as 40 mL/kg. Standard fluid, Na^+, K^+, requirement based on body surface area method is shown in Table 1.9.

Electrolyte requirements based on total fluid requirement in 24 hrs for an adult is shown in Table 1.10.

Table 1.7: Holliday - Segar formula for calculating fluid requirement

Weight	Fluid in mL 24 hours/kg	mL/kg/h	In a 24 kg child in 24 hours
First 10 kg	100	4	$100 \times 10 = 1000$ mL
Second 10 kg 11–20	50	2	$50 \times 10 = 500$ mL
Each additional 1 kg	20	1	$4 \times 20 = 80$ mL

			Total–1580 mL

Table 1.8: Fluid requirement per hour in children

Weight	Fluid in mL/h	Total volume for 24 kg child
< 10 kg	4	40
11–20 kg	2	20
> 20 kg	1	4
for each additional 1 kg		Total volume/kg = 64 mL

Table 1.9: Fluid and electrolyte requirement based on surface area/24 h

Water	1500 mL/m²/24 h
Na^+	30–50 mEq/m²/24 h
K^+	20–40 mEq/m²/24 h

Table 1.10: Electrolyte requirement based on fluid requirement

Electrolyte	Adult	Per 100 mL fluid
Sodium	100–180 mmoles	3 millimoles
Potassium	40–60 mmoles	2 millimoles
Chloride	140–240 mmoles	5 millimoles

SCENARIO 2

Calculate fluid and electrolyte requirement for a 60 kg adult?
In a patient weighing 60 kg, total fluid required in 24 hours is 60 × 40 = 2400 mL. Na required is 72 moles, K required is around 48 mmoles and chloride required is 120 mmoles. The glucose required is 100 g.
Although the amount of glucose is very low, it is the minimum amount required to ward off any ketosis, when a patient is maintained on parenteral fluids.

To find out the number of drops per minute to be given
Number of drops/minute
= *volume of liters to be infused in 24 hours × 11*
In Scenario 1 – fluid required in 24 hours is 1580 mL (1.58 L)
The number of drops/min is 1.58 × 11=18 drops/min
In Scenario 2 – fluid required in 24 hours is 2400 mL (2.4 L)
The number of drops/min is 2.4 × 11=27 drops/min
To find out the number of μ drops per minute to be given
Number of μ drops/min = Number of mL/h
In scenario 1 – the volume of fluid to be given in one hour is 64 mL,
Number of μ drops/min = 64
Interconversion between mEq/L and mg/100 mL is as follows
To convert mg/100 mL to mEq/L

$$mEq/L = \frac{mg/100\ mL \times 10 \times Valency}{Atomic\ weight}$$

Example 1: If 500 mg/100 mL of sodium chloride is to be converted into mEq/L

$$mEq/L = \frac{500 \times 10 \times 1}{58.4} = 85 \, mEq$$

To convert mEq/L to mg/100 mL

$$Mg/100 \, mL = \frac{mEq/L \times atomic \, weight}{10 \times Valency}$$

Example 2: If 85 mEq of Na Cl is to be given

$$Mg/100 \, mL = \frac{85 \times 58.46}{10 \times 1}$$

$$= 496 \, mg/100 \, mL$$
$$= 4960 \, mg/L$$
$$= around \, 5 \, g/L$$

Composition and Properties of Commonly Used IV Fluids (Table 1.12)

Sodium Chloride Solutions

1. *Isotonic saline (0.9% NaCl, Normal saline)* Normal saline contains 154 mEq/L of Na and 154 mEq/L of Cl which makes it nearly isotonic but not properly isotonic. This is because the ECF contains 140 mEq/L of Na and 106 mEq/L of Cl. Isotonic saline therefore imposes an appreciable load of chloride on kidney. Following administration, the entire volume of normal saline remains in the extracellular compartment distributed as ¾ in the interstitium and ¼ in the intravascular compartment (Table 1.11). Distribution of normal saline and Ringer's lactate is shown in Figure 1.4. Therefore one liter of normal saline will expand the plasma volume by only 250 mL. *If normal saline is used to replace the blood lost, roughly 3 times the volume should be replaced.* It is the fluid of choice in correcting ECF deficits in patients having hyponatremia, hypochloremia and metabolic alkalosis as in vomiting, gastric suction loss. Though not the ideal fluid for correcting hemorrhage, diarrhea, etc., it can be used rapidly to expand the ECF, if it is contracted.

The disadvantages of normal saline is it's relatively high sodium and chloride content which could affect a compromised renal or cardiac status. The excessive chloride content may induce or aggravate a preexisting acidosis by reducing the amount of bicarbonate.

2. *Half normal saline (0.45% NaCl)* Half normal saline contains 77 mEq of Na and 77 mEq of Cl per liter. It could also be considered to be made up of 500 mL of 0.9% NaCl and 500 mL of free water (Table 1.11). Distribution of half normal saline is shown in Figure 1.5. This free water supplements the total water deficit. It is used as a basic fluid for maintenance and to treat hypovolemic patients having hypernatremia (water deficit more than solute deficit).

3. *Hypertonic saline (3% saline)* This solution contains 513 mEq of Na and 513 mEq Cl per liter. This is used in the rapid correction of hyponatremia in conditions like SIADH.

Dextrose Solution

The commonly used dextrose solution for intravenous administration is 5% dextrose (i.e. 50 gm dextrose/liter of fluid). The dextrose in this gets metabolized to carbon dioxide and water leaving a solution physiologically equivalent to distilled water but producing no hemolysis. Two-thirds of this water moves into the ICF leaving 1/3 in ECF. Thus, 1 liter of 5% dextrose increases the intravascular volume only by 80 mL (Table 1.11). Distribution of 5% dextrose solution is shown in

Table 1.11: Distribution of commonly used IV solutions (1 liter of solution)

Solution	ICF	ECF in mL	
		Interstitial	Plasma
Isotonic saline (0.9%)	–	750	250
0.45 saline	332 mL	501	167
5% dextrose	670 mL	208	82
Colloids	–	–	1000

Table 1.12: Composition of commonly used IV fluids (mEq/L)

Solution	Dextrose	Na	K	Cl	Lactate	Ca.	others
0.9% saline		154	–	154			
0.45% saline		77	–	77	–		
5% dextrose	50 g	–		–	–		
5% DNS	50 g	154	–	154			
Ringer's lactate	–	130	4	109	28	3	
Isolyte M	50 g	40	35	40			HPO_4 15 Acetate 20
Isolyte G	50 g	63	17	150			NH_4 70
Isolyte E	50 g	140	10	103		5	Mg 3 citrate 8 Acetate 47
Isolyte P	50 g	25	20	22			HPO_4 -3 Mg 3 Acetate 23
Hemaccel	145	5	145			6.25	Gelatin 35 g
Hetastarch		154		154			Starch 60 g
5% albumin		160	2				50 g

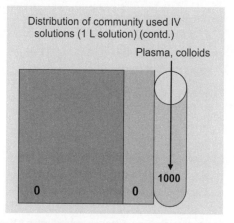

Fig. 1.2: Distribution of colloids within ICF and ECF

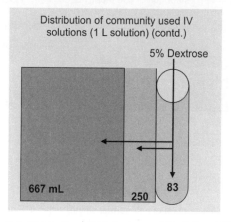

Fig. 1.3: Distribution of 5% dextrose within ICF and ECF

Figure 1.3. Dextrose solutions are primarily used to correct ICF deficits. It is not effective in correcting ECF deficits because:
1. The amount of fluid remaining in the ECF after administration of dextrose solution is minimal and hence large volumes of fluids must be administered to correct ECF deficit. This will lead to severe hyponatremia and water intoxication.

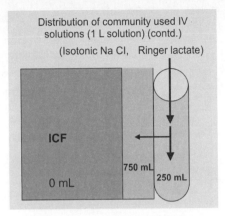

Fig. 1.4: Distribution of normal saline, Ringer's lactate within ICF and ECF

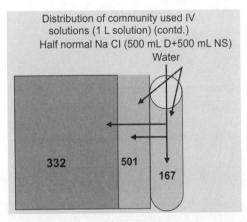

Fig. 1.5: Distribution of half normal saline, within ICF and ECF

2. When dextrose containing solutions are administered at a rate of more than 500 mL/h (i.e. glucose given at >25 g/h), it produces osmotic diuresis and worsen the ECF deficit.

Balanced Solutions

Ringer's Lactate

This is the most commonly used balanced solution. One liter of this provides 130 mEq sodium, 109 mEq Cl, 4 mEq of potassium, 3 mEq of Ca and 28 mEq of lactate. Since, the electrolyte content of Ringer is very similar to that of plasma, it is considered the most physiological solution. The lactate in this solution gets converted in the liver to bicarbonate. This solution is primarily used to correct ECF deficits especially in conditions like burns when renal function is adequate. In severe shock, there is hypoperfusion to the kidneys and liver. In such situations Ringer's lactate should not be tried because:

If the kidneys are not functioning, there can be a rise in serum potassium and will result in severe hyperkalemia. When there is hypoperfusion of the liver, the lactate does not get converted to bicarbonate and can contribute to lactic acidosis.

Colloids

Colloids are fluids containing proteins or starch molecules that remain entirely within the intravascular compartment (Fig. 1.2). This will increase the oncotic pressure inside the vessel and will draw water from the interstitium and ICF. Thus, the intravascular volume will expand. If the capillary endothelium is damaged they do not remain in circulation and leak into the interstitial space.

The commonly used colloids are:
1. Albumin
2. Dextran
3. Polygeline (Haemaccel)
4. Starch derivatives (tetrastarch, pentastarch, hetastarch).

Albumin

In normal adults albumin contributes to 80% of colloid oncotic pressure. Albumin is prepared from donor plasma and is available as 5% or 20% solution. 5% solution is osmotically and oncotically equivalent to plasma. It can be used for emergency restoration of blood volume following acute blood loss. Crystalloids should be used simultaneously to correct interstitial fluid deficit.

The definite indications are:
1. Non-hemorrhagic shock due to hypoproteinemia
2. Burn patients after the initial 24 hours if there is continuing protein loss.

3. In patients with ascites who develop hypotension after paracentesis
4. Acute/chronic liver failure
5. Protein loosing enteropathies producing hypovolemia and edema.

Disadvantages: This can produce allergic reactions and is more expensive compared to other colloids and crystalloids. Careful monitoring of patients is mandatory as they can develop pulmonary edema.

Dextran

Dextrans are polysaccharides available as low molecular weight dextran (D-40) and high molecular weight dextran (D-70). By increasing the plasma oncotic pressure, they can rapidly restore the intravascular volume. Of these D-70 is more effective because its molecular weight resembles more closely that of albumin. Though they are very effective plasma expanders, they have some disadvantages.

1. A high incidence of anaphylactic reaction
2. Dextran interferes with blood coagulation which increases the risk of bleeding. To minimize this risk it should be limited to 20 mL/kg in 24 hours
3. Interferes with cross-matching of blood.

Administration of dextran should be carefully monitored as it can cause dangerous fluid retention especially in patients with cardiac or renal disease.

Contraindications for Dextran

1. Severe bleeding disorders
2. Known hypersensitivity to dextran
3. Severe cardiac or renal failure.

Polygeline

This is a synthetic colloid made from gelatin. Its plasma volume expansion properties are similar to that of 5% albumin and continues to expand the plasma volume for a period of 24–36 hours. Although it is a good plasma expander, its hazards are similar to that of dextran in causing allergic reaction, interference with blood coagulation and circulatory overload. Because it is primarily excreted by the kidney it should not be used in renal failure.

Though colloids can rapidly increase a contracted intravascular volume, they should not be used alone because:
- Due to their high oncotic pressure they do not permit glomerular filtration.
- They do not replete the interstitial compartment which is also depleted.
- They can cause circulatory overload.

Starch (Hydroxyethyl Starch)

Composed of amylopectin (maize starch) that has been etherified with hydroxyethyl groups, mol. wt 130,000 to 450,000 daltons available in 3–6% solutions. Hydroxyethyl starch solutions have less risk of allergic reactions than dextran or gelatin solutions.

Composition of commonly used parenteral fluids is shown in Table 1.12.

KEY POINTS

- ICF contains 2/3rd of total body water.
- Only 1/12th of total body water is in the vascular compartment.
- Maintenance fluid should contain 2/3rd as free water and 1/3rd as electrolyte solution
- Colloids are distributed only in vascular compartment.
- To correct interstitial fluid deficit, normal saline, Ringer's lactate and other electrolyte solutions should be used.
- As replacement fluid for ICF, 5% dextrose is given as water cannot be administered parenterally.
- Half normal saline can also be used since 50% of this fluid distributes as free water.

Fluid Therapy in Pathological States

A Vimala

Pathological states can result in external loss of blood, body fluids or sequestration of fluids into third space.

When there is fluid loss, the volume of required fluid is calculated based on:

1. Maintenance requirement
2. Estimated loss
3. Ongoing loss.

ABNORMALITIES IN ECF VOLUME

Abnormalities in ECF volume can be a volume deficit or a volume excess. Of these two, **volume deficits** deserve special attention regarding fluid therapy.

Volume deficits are grouped into:

- Deficit of both water and electrolytes (isotonic fluid loss)
- Deficit of water alone (pure water depletion).

I. Isotonic Volume Loss

Isotonic water loss is synonymous with fluid volume deficit (FVD). Here the fluid loss is similar to the ECF and therefore, the osmolality of the ECF is not altered. As a result there is no shift of fluid from the ICF and deficit is localized to the ECF alone and clinical features seen would be those of ECF volume depletion alone. Within the ECF, it is intravascular volume that gets depleted first followed by the interstitial compartment.

Whenever, there is isotonic fluid deficit, one must look for postural hypotension, postural tachycardia as these are the earliest signs of fluid depletion.

Symptoms and signs of volume deficit depends on the fluid compartment that has lost fluid.

1. Signs of Intravascular Volume Depletion

Depending on the degree of blood loss, signs and symptoms will develop. Classification is shown in Table 2.1.

2. Signs of Interstitial Fluid Volume Depletion

1. Dry tongue with longitudinal furrowing
2. Decreased skin turgor noted best over the forehead and sternum
3. Sunken eyes.

Etiologic factors are:

1. Blood loss — Trauma, surgery, APH, PPH, GI bleed
2. Loss of gastrointestinal fluid — vomiting, diarrhea, gastric suction, fistulae, drainage tubes.

Table 2.1: Classification based on blood volume loss 70 kg man

Variable	Class I	Class II	Class III	Class IV
Blood loss, mL (% blood volume)	< 750	750–1500	1500–2000	> 2000
	(< 15%)	(15–30%)	(30–40%)	(> 40%)
Pulse rate	Normal	> 100	> 120	> 140
Blood pressure	Normal	Normal	Decreased	Decreased
Respiratory rate	Normal	20–30	30–35	> 35
Urine output	Normal	20–30 mL/hr	5–1 5 mL/hr	Anuric
Mental status	anxious	anxious	Confused	Confused lethargic
Response to fluid bolus	Yes	Yes	Transient	No

{Adapted from American College of Surgeons, Committee on Trauma: Advanced Trauma Life Support for Doctors, 6th ed. 1997, p 98.}

3. Polyuria – diuretics, renal failure, diabetes mellitus, etc.
4. Internal sequestration (3rd space loss) – massive ascites, Paralytic ileus, cellulitis.
5. Burns.

II. Pure Water Depletion

In pure water loss or if water is lost more than sodium the ECF osmolality will increase and to achieve osmotic equilibrium water will move from the cell to the interstitium and cells become dehydrated. The clinical signs and symptoms are due to cellular dehydration.

Etiological Factors

1. Reduced water intake (restricted access to water, defective thirst, cerebrovascular accident)
2. Sweating (fever, heat stroke)
3. Loss through lungs – Hyperventilation, tracheostomy, fever.

Sweat is hypotonic fluid (1 liter contains 40 mmol of sodium and 50 mmol of chloride). Excessive sweating can cause water depletion unless corrected by fluids. In fever there is increased evaporative loss of water and additional requirement for rise in temperature should be given. In fever there is 10–15% increase in maintenance fluid requirement.

Additional requirement is calculated as 250 mL/day for each degree centigrade above 37° C and for every 1.6°F above 98.4°F.

> **Example:** In a patient with a temperature of 100°F, additional fluid requirement = 250 × 1.6 = 400 mL (Evaporative water loss is pure water and should be replaced with water orally or 5% dextrose through parenteral route).

Signs of ICF Depletion

Thirst is the cardinal symptom of ICF depletion. The increase in ECF osmolality stimulates thirst. If the fluid loss is not checked at this point, the patient develops intracellular dehydration resulting in cerebral manifestations like altered sensorium, convulsions and coma in severe cases.

Parenteral Correction of Fluid Volume Deficit

In certain conditions, oral rehydration cannot be employed fully. Here parenteral correction should be done. Before correction, the body fluid requirement should be calculated by carefully assessing the vital signs. To this the maintenance requirement and the ongoing losses should be added. The ideal solution for initiating correction of fluid volume deficit is *normal saline*. Once urine production is ensured the remaining deficit can be corrected by using *Ringer's lactate*.

The advantage of giving lactate is that lactate is converted to bicarbonate which could correct the acidosis.

In cases of massive fluid loss with severe hypotension, the primary aim is to rapidly increase the blood pressure.

In this situation, normal saline along with simultaneous administration of colloids can rapidly elevate the blood pressure. But this requires careful monitoring. After correcting the blood pressure, further fluid therapy is best guided by urine output (> 30 mL/h) and central venous pressure maintained at 8 cm of water. After the initial administration of fluid, if urine output is inadequate, it indicates impending acute renal failure.

The composition and volume of fluid loss will decide the appropriate replacement solution. The composition of various body fluids is shown in Table 2.2.

Table 2.2: Composition of various body fluids

Common losses	Body fluid	Composition (mEq/L)			
		Na^+	K^+	Cl^-	HCO_3^-
Sweating (fever)	Sweat	20–50	5–10	45–55	–
Gastrointestinal					
Nasogastric tube, vomiting	Gastric	40–80	5–15	90–130	
Biliary fistula	Biliary	130–150	5–10	80–120	30–40
Pancreatic fistula	Pancreatic	120–140	5–10	60–90	90–110
Duodenal tube, fistula	Duodenal	130–140	5–10	70–90	0–50
Ileostomy, fistula	Ileal	100–140	5–10	80–110	20–30
Diarrhea, colostomy	Colon	50–70	20–40	30–50	20–30

Na^+, sodium; K^+, potassium; Cl^-, chloride; HCO_3^-, bicarbonate

Parameters monitored are
1. Sensorium
2. Vital signs
3. Central venous pressure (CVP)
4. Pulmonary capillary wedge pressure (PCWP).
   a. Sensorium—Improvement in sensorium indicate correction of ICF volume.
   b. Vital signs—Decrease in pulse rate, decrease in heart rate, increase in blood pressure and decrease in respiratory rate are pointers of ECF volume correction.
   c. Central venous pressure (CVP)—This measures the pressure inside the right atrium and normally is around 5–8 cm of water. This provides information about vascular volume, vascular tone, and effectiveness of pumping action. CVP should be monitored at half hourly intervals. A single value has no significance. The direction of progression of CVP should be monitored. If increase in CVP parallels the changes in blood pressure. It indicates fluid deficit and need for adequate replacement. Even after large volume of fluid administration, if CVP remains low, this may suggest ongoing loss.

Fallacies in interpretation of CVP
   i. CVP is influenced by compliance of veins and ventricles, both of which are decreased in hypovolemia. The excessive venoconstriction resulting from sympathetic activation may produce falsely high CVP reading.
   ii. Use of vasopressors like dopamine may give a higher CVP.
   iii. Conditions like cardiac tamponade or tension pneumothorax may give a false high reading.
   Causes for changes in central venous pressure (CVP) is shown in Table 2.3.

Table 2.3: Changes in central venous pressure

Low CVP	High CVP
Low circulating volume	Fluid overload
Vasodialatation	Cardiac failure
	Vasopressors, vasoconstriction

Table 2.4: Commonly used electrolytes content in mEq/g of salt

Salt	mEq/g
Sodium chloride	17
Sodium bicarbonate	12
Potassium chloride	13
Calcium carbonate	2 0

d. Pulmonary Capillary Wedge Pressure (PCWP)–Detailed hemodynamic monitoring by PCWP is not usually done. It is done in certain situations like
  • Hypovolemia complicating other forms of shock like cardiogenic shock, septic shock
  • Poor myocardial function
  • Persistently high CVP with inadequate volume
  • Patient developing pulmonary edema
  • While using vasopressors.
    Normal PCWP is 6–12 cm of water and measures the pressure in the left atrium.

Route of Fluid Administration

Oral Fluids

This is the best way of administering fluids. This is the most physiological route and replace electrolytes minerals and nutrients adequately. There is no danger of infection or fluid overload. Hence, parenteral fluid therapy should be resorted to only if oral therapy is not feasible.

Oral replacement of electrolytes can be given as normal food supplements with added electrolytes. The content of Na in mEq/g is shown in Table 2.4.

SCENARIO 3

A 45-year-old female of weight 50 kg is admitted with diarrhea. She has a blood pressure of 90/60 mm Hg, pulse rate of 110/min, dry tongue with normal furrowing, and has normal sensorium. She is unable to tolerate fluids orally. Her urine output is 30 mL/h.

Fluid requirement is calculated as follows:

Fluid requirement = maintenance fluid + 50% of deficit + ongoing loss

Maintenance fluid (40 mL/kg) = 2000 mL

Maintenance fluid should consist 66% as free water and 34% as electrolyte solution.

1320 mL as 5% dextrose and 680 mL of fluid containing Na and K.

Na and K requirement can also be calculated as follows:

Na requirement = 3 mmol for every 100 mL = 60 mmol

K requirement = 2 mmol for every 100 mL = 40 mmol

Cl requirement = 5 mmol for every 100 mL = 100 mmol

1000 mL of half normal saline contains 77 mmol Na and 77 mmol Cl. To give 60 mmols, half normal saline required is 780 mL.

K can be given as 20 mL of KCl (1 mL = 2 mmol)

Deficit Correction

Hypotension, tachycardia indicate moderate hypovolemia and fluid deficit is 60 mL/kg, in this lady, 60 × 50 = 3000 mL.

50% i.e. 1500 mL has to be replaced in the first 24 hours.

Since, this is ECF volume depletion, normal saline is the fluid of choice.

Ongoing Loss This patient had 5 bouts of loose stools.

For each diarrheal stool, 200 mL fluid has to be replaced.

Since fluid lost contains bicarbonate and potassium, sodium bicarbonate and potassium also has to be replaced.

K containing fluid has to be infused after ensuring that urine output and renal parameters are normal. This lady had normal serum creatinine and had passed urine. Ongoing loss can be replaced as Ringer's lactate

Fluid on the first day = 1320 mL of 5% dextrose + 680 mL of half normal saline +1500 mL of normal saline + 1000 mL of Ringer's lactate. 5 mL of KCl can be added to each pint of normal saline and 1 pint of half normal saline.

Resuscitation Fluid Therapy in Burns

Different formulas are available for calculating fluid requirement in burns.

Some formulas are shown in Table 2.5.

Table 2.5: Resuscitation formulas

Formula	Fluid in first 24 hours	Crystalloid in second 24 hours	Colloid in second 24 hours
Parkland	RL at 4 mL/kg per percentage burn	20–60% estimated plasma volume	Titrated to urinary output of 30 mL/h
Evans	NS at 1 mL/kg per percentage burn, 2000 mL 5% dextrose, and colloid at 1 mL/kg per percentage burn	50% of first 24-hours volume plus 2000 mL D5W	50% of first 24 hours volume
Slater	RL at 2 L/24 h plus fresh frozen plasma at 75 mL/kg/24 h		
Brooke	RL at 1.5 mL/kg per percentage burn, colloid at 0.5 mL/kg burn, and 2000 mL D5W	50% of first 24 hours volume plus 2000 mL D5W	50% of first 24 hours volume
Modified brooke	RL at 2 mL/kg per percentage burn		

KEY POINTS

- Fluid therapy is based on physiological distribution of water and composition of body fluid lost.
- Assess maintenance requirement and replace in 24 hours.
- ECF fluid deficit and excess corrected based on clinical signs of hypovolemia and fluid overload.
- 50% of fluid deficit is corrected in first 24 hours and the remaining in next 24 hours.
- Ongoing loss has to be replaced and the fluid should be similar in composition to the fluid lost.

EARLY GOAL-DIRECTED THERAPY

The surviving sepsis campaign 2008 guidelines define early goal directed therapy in first 6 hours of sepsis. Sepsis syndrome and it's sequelae are important causes of morbidity and mortality. The pathogenesis of this entity is very complex and will not be discussed here. Early detection and aggressive management can significantly reduce mortality from sepsis. Treatment is mainly directed towards elimination of organism and toxin. With the institution of early goal directed therapy in early hours of sepsis, the course can be altered . There is a reduction in mortality.

For whom should we consider "**Early goal directed therapy?**"

INDICATIONS

1. Suspected infection
2. SIRS
   Diagnosis of SIRS is based on the presence of two or more of the following:
   a. Temperature > 38°C or < 36°C
   b. Pulse > 90 beats/min
   c. Respirations > 20 breaths/min or arterial partial pressure of carbon dioxide ($PaCO_2$) < 32 mm Hg
   d. White blood cell count > 12,000 or < 4000 cells/mm^3 or > 10% bands

3. Evidence of hypoperfusion—systolic blood pressure less than 90 mm Hg after 20–30 mL/kg fluid challenge or a lactic acid level more than 4 mmol/L.

OBJECTIVES OF EARLY GOAL-DIRECTED THERAPY

- To normalize preload and blood pressure
- To prevent tissue hypoxia by matching oxygen delivery with consumption.

Specific goals for normalizing preload and pressure are:

1. To maintain a central venous pressure of 8–12 mm Hg in patients not on ventilator and 12–15 mm Hg in those who are mechanically ventilated or have decreased ventricular compliance
2. To achieve a mean arterial pressure (MAP) 65 mm Hg or greater
3. Central venous or mixed venous oxygen saturation 70% or greater
4. Urine output of 0.5 mL/kg/h or greater.

Step 1: To normalize preload and blood pressure

The first step in goal-directed therapy is to provide a proper filling pressure to ensure adequate cardiac preload. This is achieved by maintaining a central venous pressure of 8–12 mm Hg in patients not on ventilator and 12–15 mm Hg in those who are mechanically ventilated or have decreased ventricular compliance. Fluids have to be administered parenterally to achieve target CVP. Crystalloids or colloids can be used. Normal saline or Ringer's lactate is the fluid of first choice. As soon as hypoperfusion is recognized, 1000 mL of normal saline or 500 mL of colloids have to be infused over 30 minutes.

Care must be taken to avoid fluid overload and pulmonary edema. Patients with cardiac dysfunction and acute kidney injury are at high risk for *fluid overload and pulmonary edema.* Though Lactic acidosis can occur with infusion of Ringer's lactate this is not usually observed.

Parameters monitored during fluid challenge

Parameters	Positive response
i. Heart rate	Decrease in heart rate
ii. Blood pressure	Increase in blood pressure
iii. Capillary filling	Capillary refill
iv. Temperature of skin	increase in skin temperature
v. Change in mental status	improvement in sensorium
vi. Urine output	0.5 mL to 1 mL/kg/h or greater

Adequate blood pressure is taken as a mean arterial pressure between 60 and 90 mm Hg.

Even after attaining the target CVP as mentioned above, if the mean arterial pressure of 65 mm Hg is not attained proceed to step 2.

Step 2: Vasopressors are indicated

Norepinephrine or dopamine are considered first-line agents.

1. **Norepinephrine:** Norepinephrine is a mixed alpha and beta agonist and has only minimal beta$_2$ activity.
   Action—It increases cardiac output, systemic vascular resistance and also improves GFR and urine output.
   Dose is 0.5 to 3 µg/kg/min.
2. **Dopamine:** It is the drug of choice for patients who are unresponsive to adequate volume expansion. Dopamine is primarily an alpha, beta$_1$, and dopaminergic agonist.
   Dopamine is no longer used as an agent to increase renal perfusion if MAP is normal.
   Side effects are related to the dose. Dosages greater than 20 µg/kg/min produce persistent tachycardia, decreased partial pressure of arterial oxygen (PaO$_2$) and increased pulmonary artery occlusion pressure. It can precipitate tachyarrythmias, GI bleeding and induce acute lung injury.
3. **Phenylephrine:** Phenylephrine is a selective alpha$_1$-agonist, effective in restoring perfusion in patients with septic shock refractory to dopamine or dobutamine . This drug

increases systemic vascular resistance without significant changes in cardiac output. Rarely, it can produce reflex bradycardia or suppression in cardiac output. This may be used in patients with tachyarrhytmias where other agents are contraindicated.

4. **Epinephrine:** Epinephrine is a very potent mixed alpha and beta agonist. Epinephrine infusion is also associated with increased oxygen consumption, increased systemic lactate concentrations and decreased splanchnic blood flow. Hence, it is currently recommended only for those patients who are unresponsive to other vasopressors.

5. **Vasopressin:** Vasopressin is a naturally occurring non-apeptide that is synthesized as a large prohormone in the hypothalamus. Vasopressin should not be used as the sole initial therapy for refractory septic shock

   Once preload and pressure are normalized, the next focus is on oxygen delivery.

   Goal — to maintain a SpO_2 saturation of 95% or the patient's baseline in the case of underlying lung disease.

   The best index for assessing oxygen delivery is by measuring mixed venous saturation. The target is a mixed venous saturation ($ScvO_2$) greater than 70%. If $ScvO_2$ is less than 70% proceed to step 3.

Step 3

Decrease in oxygen delivery occurs due to

a. Reduction in hemoglobin as a result of marrow suppression and dilution with crystalloid fluids that are infused.

b. hypoperfusion can be a result of global and distributive changes in both systemic blood flow and microvasculature.

To increase hemoglobin, packed red cell transfusions can be given to attain target Hb 11 gm and PCV27 to 30%. The arterial oxygen saturation should be optimized with non-rebreather oxygen delivery or intubation, as needed.

After attaining target hemoglobin or PCV if $ScvO_2$ is not attained.

Ionotropic agents that can increase cardiac contractility and cardiac output can be used to increase oxygen delivery.

Ionotropic Agents

Dobutamine — Dobutamine is a mixed alpha and beta-agonist. Starting dose is 2 µg/kg/min and can be increased to a maximum of 28 µg/kg/min.

Dosing of vasoactive therapy

Drug	Dosage
Dobutamine	5-1 5 µg/kg/min
Dopamine	2-20 µg/kg/min
Epinephrine	5-20 µg/min
Norepinephrine	5-20 µg/min
Phenylephrine	2-20 µg/min

The most important bad prognostic factor is inadequate ventilation. Inadequate ventilation is indicated by respiratory rate greater than 30 breaths per minute, irrespective of arterial oxygenation.

Indications for Mechanical Ventilation

1. Hypercapnia,
2. Persistent hypoxemia,
3. Airway compromise and
4. Profound acidosis.

In acute lung injury current recommendations are to maintain transalveolar pressures measured as plateau pressures below 35 cm H_2O with increasing end-expiratory pressure and low tidal volumes (6 mL/kg).

Patients with sepsis syndrome can develop moderate to severe acidosis, hyperglyc emia and adrenal insufficiency.

Correction of Acidosis with Bicarbonate Supplementation

It is indicated only in severe acidemia - pH < 7.0, as there may be a paradoxical decrease in intracellular pH as a result of diffusion of soluble CO_2 across the cell membrane.

Glycemic Control

Aim is to achieve a blood glucose concentration between 130 and 150 mg. Insulin should be given intravenously monitoring blood glucose levels 2 hourly. Patients receiving intravenous insulin should simultaneously receive some form of glucose as a calorie source to minimize the risk of hypoglycemia.

Adrenal Insufficiency

Patients with severe sepsis can develop glucocorticoid and mineralocorticoid deficiency .This is corrected with Hydrocortisone which should be administered intravenously 200–300 mg/day in 4 divided doses or as a continuous infusion.

Duration of treatment is 7 days. If another form of corticosteroid other than hydrocortisone is used, then fludrocortisone at a dose of 50 µg/day should be added for mineralocorticoid effect.

Activated protein C which was used has now been withdrawn.

Prophylactic Measures

1. **Unfractionated or low-molecular-weight heparin** for prophylaxis against deep venous thrombosis.
2. Histamine 2 (H_2) blocker or proton pump inhibitor for gastric ulcer prophylaxis.

KEY POINTS

Initial Six Hours

Investigations for identifying the pathogen and source of infection.

- Blood, urine, and other appropriate cultures (cerebrospinal fluid, abscess drainage, catheter tip, tissue, sputum) before starting empiric antimicrobial therapy.
- Appropriate imaging studies guided by patient's clinical status.
- Removal of the potentially infected foreign bodies like catheters, vascular access.

Treatment

- Initiate fluid resuscitation with crystalloid or colloid to achieve central venous pressure of 12 mm Hg (or 15 mm Hg if intubated).
- Add dopamine or norepinephrine for persistent hypotension (mean arterial pressure < 65 mm Hg).
- Dobutamine therapy for low cardiac output in the face of adequate filling pressures.
- Vasopressin, epinephrine in refractory hypotension.
- Packed red cell transfusions to increase O_2 delivery.
- Maintain glycemic control with a target blood glucose level between 130 and 150 mg/dL.
- Consider therapy with hydrocortisone for patients with continued hypotension despite adequate fluid resuscitation, vasopressors and acidosis correction.

All interventions should be undertaken simultaneously and initiated within 1 hour after making a presumptive diagnosis of sepsis.

3

Sodium Homeostasis and Renal Regulation of Sodium

A Vimala

OVERVIEW

Sodium is the predominant extracellular cation. Kidney is the main organ regulating the excretion of sodium. ECF volume is determined by the sodium content. Sodium balance is mainly maintained by regulating the excretion of sodium by the kidney. Normally 99% of sodium that is filtered by the glomeruli is reabsorbed. Sodium homeostasis is maintained by regulating excretion of final 1% of filtered sodium. This small change is equivalent to addition or removal of one liter of fluid daily to the ECF volume. To maintain constant sodium balance, sodium intake should be equal to the sodium excretion in the urine. If the daily intake of sodium is 150 millimoles, then 150 millimoles is lost in urine to maintain Na balance. When sodium content increases the ECF volume expands and this is sensed by receptors situated in the arterial and local venous channels. They send signals through renal nerves, hormones and physical changes to the kidneys to increase the excretion of sodium and maintain sodium balance. Similarly, when ECF volume contracts reabsorption of sodium will increase and ECF volume will be maintained.

RENAL HANDLING OF SODIUM

Normally around 27000 millimoles of sodium is filtered by the glomeruli. Of the filtered sodium more than 99% is reabsorbed and only 0.5–1% is excreted. Maintenance of Sodium Chloride (Na Cl) is absolutely necessary for normal functioning of cells. The glomeruli and tubules interact to maintain Na Cl balance. There are two important physiological mechanisms that maintain the renal blood flow (RBF) and GFR within narrow limits. Glomeruli respond to tubules by tubuloglomerular feedback and tubules respond to glomeruli by glomerulotubular balance. When GFR increases or decreases, parallel changes in proximal tubular reabsorbtion occurs.

CONTROL OF PROXIMAL TUBULAR SODIUM REABSORPTION

Glomerulotubular Balance (GTB)

When GFR increases proximal tubular reabsorption of sodium will also increase. This will minimize the variations in fractional proximal fluid absorption. Factors controlling GTB are:

1. Peritubular Capillary Oncotic Pressure

When the GFR increases there will be increasing filtration fraction causing an increase in the oncotic pressure in the postglomerular peritubular capillaries. This will decrease the absolute rate of fluid reabsorption. Other factors controlling the proximal tubular reabsorption are: catecholomines, parathyroid hormone, angiotensin, thyroid hormone, corticosteroids and nitric oxide.

2. Tubuloglomerular Feedback

This is an important mechanism by which GFR is regulated. This is achieved by renin-angiotensin mechanism (Fig. 3.1).

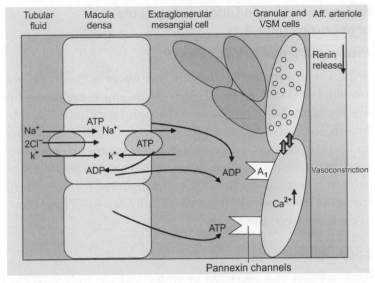

Fig. 3.1: Tubuloglomerular feedback

Macular densa is a collection of densely packed cells at the junction of thick ascending limb and early distal tubule. This is set at an angle between afferent arteriole and efferent arteriole. Macular densa senses rapidly changes in the composition of fluid flowing through thick ascending limb (TAL). Increased Na Cl delivery to distal nephron is an indicator of increased GFR whereas low sodium and chloride delivery is an indicator of decreased GFR. Macular densa senses the Na Cl by the apical Na⁻k⁻ 2Cl for transport. Signaling molecules are released. This brings appropriate changes in GFR. This is based on purinergic signalling. ATP is released through pannexin channels from cells. Extracellular ATP is converted to Adenosine. This binds to Adenosine A^1 receptors on extraglomerular mesangial cells. This triggers a rise in intracellular Ca levels. The calcium signal is propagated through gap junctions of adjacent cells including granular cells of juxtaglomerular apparatus and vascular smooth muscle cells of afferent arteriole and decrease release of renin. This decreases GFR.

Sodium Handling in Different Segments of Nephron (Table 3.1)

Proximal Convoluted Tubules (PCT)

In PCT, reabsorbtion of sodium and water is isosmotic and around 18000 millimoles (2/3rd) of sodium is reabsorbed in this segment. Na enters the cell through apical membrane by two mechanisms, this is coupled to reabsorption of chloride and secretion of H^+ ions. Second mechanism is independent entry of Sodium. For these two mechanisms the driving force is electrochemical gradient. The driving force for the sodium transport from the cell to the blood is by Na^+K^+ATPase pump in the basolateral membrane.

Loop of Henle

Reabsorption and secretion of water and electrolytes occurs as the filtrate traverses the loop of Henle. The dissociation of salt and water absorption by the loop of Henle is responsible for the capacity of the kidney to concentrate or dilute the urine. The descending limb of loop of Henle is permeable only to water and is impermeable to electrolytes and as a result osmolality of tubular fluid increases progressively and the maximum osmolality of 1200–1400 milliosmoles is achieved at the tip of the descending limb. The ascending limb of loop of Henle is permeable only to electrolytes and is impermeable to water. In the ascending limb 50% of sodium is reabsorbed via luminal $Na^+K^+2Cl^-$ cotransporter and the driving force is

Table 3.1: Sodium reabsorption by the kidney

Nephron site	Na reabsorption	Remaining	
PCT	18000	9000	150/L
Ascending limb of loop of Henle	6000	3000	45/L
DCT	1600	1400	100/L
Cortical collecting duct	800	600	100/L
Medullary collecting duct	450	150	150/L

by Na⁺K⁺ATPase situated in basolateral membrane. Of 3000 millimoles of sodium reabsorbed, 1500 millimoles of sodium is reabsorbed via Na⁺K⁺2Cl⁻ cotransporter and the remaining 1500 millimoles of sodium is reabsorbed passively via paracellular path way. The exit of Na⁺ and Cl⁻ is an energy requiring process against a concentration gradient and the driving force is by Na⁺K⁺ATPase. Reabsorption is stimulated by ADH and inhibited by diuretics (Fig. 3.2).

Distal Convoluted Tubule (DCT)

In DCT sodium is reabsorbed along with chloride and is sparingly permeable to water.

Collecting Duct

Sodium reabsorption is linked to chloride reabsorption and to secretion of potassium and H⁺ions. Sodium channel is stimulated by increase in distal blood flow. This is also mediated through aldosterone. In the medulla along with

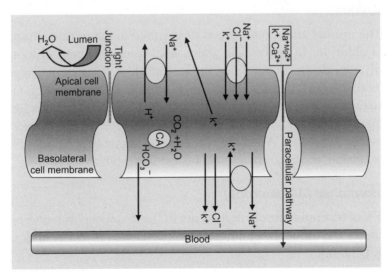

Fig. 3.2: Na reabsorption in proximal tubule

sodium balance, concentration of urine and ammonium excretion occurs. Atrial natriuretic factor acts for regulation of sodium reabsorption.

Factors Regulating Na+ Excretion

Maintenance of Sodium Chloride (Na Cl) is absolutely necessary for normal functioning of cells. The glomeruli and tubules interact to maintain Na Cl balance. There are two important physiological mechanisms that maintain the renal blood flow (RBF) and GFR within narrow limits. Glomeruli respond to tubules by tubuloglomerular feedback and tubules respond to glomeruli by glomerulotubular balance.

ECF Volume

When ECF volume is contracted urine is free of Na^+ and Cl^- and when expanded urine Na will be increased. Thus, there are no normal values for urinary Na and Cl and should be interpreted relative to the fluid status of the patient and dietary intake.

Anions

The normal anion reabsorbed or excreted along with sodium is chloride. In pathologic states like vomiting there is loss of chloride in gastric juice hence only less chloride will be available for reabsorption along with sodium. Sodium is reabsorbed with other anion HCO_3 and this generates metabolic alkalosis. The quantity of bicarbonate delivered to the kidney is also increased. When the reabsorptive capacity of tubules is exceeded, the bicarbonate will be lost with sodium in urine.

Hormones (Aldosterone)

5% of sodium reabsorption occurs in the distal nephron and is under the influence of aldosterone [Discussed in detail under K balance].

Angiotensin 11

Angiotensin is released from juxtaglomerular apparatus. Hypovolemia, low renal perfusion pressure, increased sympathetic activity and rise in beta adrenergic agonists will stimulate angiotensin release. Angiotensin 11 will increase the reabsorption of sodium in PCT along with water.

This leads to increase in chloride concentration in the lumen which is passively reabsorbed. Angiotensin 11 is a powerful efferent arteriolar constrictor and will increase the intraglomerular pressure and increases GFR. Increased filtrate in the PCT lumen will increase the reabsorption of Na and solute.

KEY POINTS

- Reabsorption of Na is isoosmotic in Proximal tubule.
- 50% of Na is reabsorbed via luminal $Na^+K^+2Cl^-$ cotransporter.
- In collecting duct sodium reabsorption is linked to chloride reabsorption and to secretion of potassium and H^+ ions.

Hyponatremia

A Vimala

OVERVIEW

Sodium (Na) is the most abundant and important cation in the extracellular fluid. Content of ECF sodium determines ECF volume plasma osmolality is mainly determined by Sodium. Normal serum sodium varies from 135 to 145 mmol/L. Normal plasma osmolality ranges from 285–295 milliosmoles/kg of water. Decrease in plasma osmolality is always associated with increase in cell volume. This is responsible for the symptoms and signs of hyponatremia and also for the complications that arise during inappropriate rapid correction. Hyponatremia is the most common electrolyte abnormality encountered in clinical practice, occurring in up to 15 to 30% of both acutely and chronically ill hospitalized patients. The reported incidence in intensive care unit varies from 40–50%. Sodium deficit and rate of rise in sodium concentration with administration of sodium containing infusates can be calculated based on formulae. Guidelines are available for the management of hyponatremia.

Milestones

Diagnosis of hyponatremia was possible with the introduction of flame photometer by Barnes, Richardson, and Berry in 1945 after the Second World War. Consequences of salt depletion in normal man was described by Marriot in 1947. Peter et al described hyponatremia with salt wasting in 1950.

Cerebral salt wasting syndrome as a cause of hyponatremia was identified in 1952. Leaf et al noted in 1953 that ADH infusion can result in salt wasting and hyponatremia. This led to the use of V_2 receptor antagonists in the treatment of hyponatremia. Conivaptan was approved for the management of hyponatremia by FDA in 2004.

What is Hyponatremia?

Definition

Hyponatremia is defined as serum sodium < 135 mmol/L and severe hyponatremia when sodium is lower than 125 mmol/L in children and 120 mmol/L in adults. Main determinant of ECF osmolality is sodium and reduction in sodium is always associated with low osmolality. "True Hyponatremia, is always hypoosmolar".

There are two conditions where low sodium can be associated with normal or high osmolality and will be discussed below.

When the plasma osmolality is normal or high, other causes should be excluded. Based on plasma osmolality hyponatremia can be classified into, hyperosmolar, isoosmolar and hypoosmolar hyponatremia (Fig. 4.1).

WHAT CAUSES HYPONATREMIA?

Sodium (Na) is expressed as concentration in mmol/L. ie. sodium (mmol)/Water (Liters) = mmol/L.Hyponatremia is not always due to loss of sodium and loss of water. Low Na does not always mean true reduction in sodium, caused by loss of Na and volume.

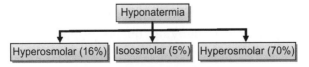

Fig. 4.1: Classification of hyponatremia

Low Na can be associated with low, normal or high ECF volume.

> **Example 1:** 140 mmol of Na dissolved in 1000 mL of H_2O gives Na concentration of 140 mmol/L.
> 140 mmol/L is dissolved in 1500 mL i.e. 500 ml in excess, Na will be =140/1500 × 1000 = 92 mmol/L/L, Here the reduction in Na is due to excess of water but there is no actual change in sodium.
> Na dissolved in 1000 mL of H_2O = 140 mmol/L/L. If there is loss of 52 mmol of sodium and 200 mL of water from the above solution, new Na concentration will be 88/800 = 110 mmol/L. Here there is loss of sodium and water but sodium is lost more than water, giving rise to a reduction in Na.
> Thus, it can be understood that serum sodium can decrease when there is sodium deficit, increase in water, or loss of sodium more than water.

Hyperosmolar Hyponatremia

In plasma, Osmolality is contributed by glucose, urea, sodium and potassium and is calculated using the formula

$$P_{osm} = \frac{Glucose\,(mg/dL)}{18} + \frac{Blood\,urea\,(mg/dL)}{6} + 2\,[Na^+\,(mmol/L) + K^+\,(mmol/L)]$$

2 × (Na + K), because Na^+ and K^+ exist as NaCl and KCl. when it dissociates, it dissociates into two osmotically active particles.

Since, Na is the most important electrolyte determining osmolality the above formula for calculating osmolality can be simplified as = 2 × plasma Na i.e. if Na is 140 mmol/L, osmolality is 140 × 2 = 280 mosmoles/kg.

Plasma concentration of K is very low (3.5–5 mmol/L), Hence, it is not considered in the simple formula.

Mechanism of Hyperosmolar Hyponatremia

Physical principle underlying this is osmosis. When two solutions of different concentrations are separated by a semi-permeable membrane, water moves from low concentration (low osmolality) to high concentration (high osmolality) to attain osmotic equilibrium. This phenomenon is **osmosis**.

Normal plasma osmolality is 287 to 295 mosmoles/kg. If 50 mmoles of osmotically active solutes are added, the ECF osmolality will increase from normal osmolaliy of 290 to 340 osmoles. Osmosis takes place and fluid will shift from low osmolality to high osmolality. A new osmotic equilibrium will be attained in the ICF and ECF.

Do All Osmotically Active Solutes Shift Water to the Same Extent?

Osmolality and Tonicity

Substances which are capable of shifting water by increasing the osmolality are *hyperosmolar and hypertonic.*

But osmotically active substances like urea can enter the cell freely and a new equilibration takes place between the ICF and ECF solute. Hence, efflux of water from the cell does not occur. Think of a solute like sodium or glucose which cannot enter the cell. The new osmotic equilibrium will be achieved by **efflux of water** from the cell to the ECF. So these particles which are impermeable to the cell, exert an oncotic pressure and are described as hypertonic solutes. Thus, it can be understood that, *all hypertonic solutes are hyperosmolar but all hyperosmolar solutes need not be hypertonic.* Glucose is a hyperosmolar hypertonic solute, but urea is hyperosmolar but not a hypertonic solute.

Other solutes like mannitol, Sorbitol, radiocontrast agents etc can also increase the osmolality and shift water to ECF. This will dilute the sodium and give a low value.

Case History 1

What is the difference in water movement between two patients, patient 1 who has a plasma urea of 120 mg% and patient 2 with a plasma glucose of 360 mg% ?

As seen in the formula, increase in glucose and urea will increase the osmolality of plasma.

The osmolality due to glucose is 360/18 = 20 and due to urea is 120/6 = 20 osmoles/kg. Thus, both glucose and urea will increase the osmolality of plasma from 290 to 310 mosmoles/kg. Hence, both should shift water from ICF to ECF.

What Happens When Urea Increases?

When urea increases in the ECF, the osmolality of plasma and ECF will increase initially. Urea is a freely diffusible solute and hence equilibrates quickly between ECF and ICF. The osmolality of ECF and ICF will be increased to the same degree. So there will be no net movement of water from ICF to ECF

With increase in urea by 20 millimoles, new osmotic equilibrium will be achieved at 290 (Fig. 4.2).

What Happens When Glucose in Plasma Increases?

When glucose concentration increases in plasma, the osmolality of ECF increases, Glucose is not a freely diffusible solute

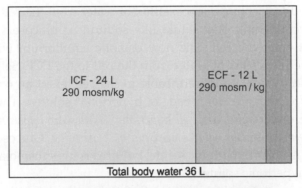

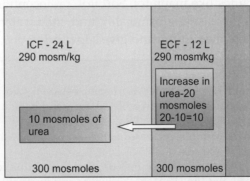

Fig. 4.2: Changes in ECF and ICF osmolality with urea

and does not enter the cell. So ECF osmolality will increase and ICF osmolality will not change. So to attain osmotic equilibrium between ICF and ECF, water moves from ICF to ECF. The increase in water in the ECF will dilute the solutes and Na in ECF will be low. This is described as translocational hyponatremia.

When 20 mosmoles of Glucose is added to ECF, the osmolality of ECF increased from 290–310 mosmoles. Glucose is impermeant and hence ICF osmolality didl not change. To attain osmotic equilibrium, water shifted from ICF to ECF (Fig. 4.3).

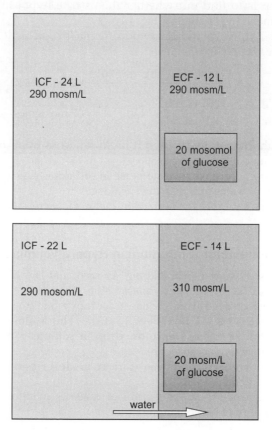

Fig. 4.3: Translocational hyponatremia (hyperosmolar hyponatremia)

Case History 2

A 60-year-old diabetic woman is admitted with alteration of sensorium. Systemic examination was unremarkable
Laboratory parameters are as follows:

Parameter	Value
RBS	540 mg%
Urea	54 mg%
Sodium	132 mmol/L

Diagnosis—Diabetes mellitus and hyponatremia
What is the cause for hyponatremia?
First step is to find out whether this is true hypoosmolar or hyperosmolar hyponatremia (Fig. 4.4)
Step 1: Is it true hypoosmolar hyponatremia (hypotonic)
Calculate Osmolality –

$$P_{osm} = \frac{G\ (mg/dL)}{18} + \frac{BU\ (mg/dL)}{6} + 2 \times (Na + K)$$

$$= \frac{540}{18} + \frac{54}{6} + 2 \times (130 + 4) = 307\ mosmoles/Kg,$$

Since the osmolality is high it is classified as hyperosmolar (translocational) hyponatremia.
Step 2: To find out whether decrease in sodium is due to dilution from shift of water from ICF to ECF alone.

We have to apply the correction factor for increase in plasma glucose:

Correction Factor for Sodium in Hyperglycemia

For increase in glucose from 100 mg, for every 100 mg, Na drops by 1.6 mmoles/L till 400 mg and 2.4 mmol/L above 400 mg.

When glucose is 540 mg, change in sodium = $(3 \times 1.6) + (1.4 \times 2.4)$ = 8.2 expected Na will be $(140–8.2)$ = 131.8. This is almost similar to the obtained value. Hence the drop in sodium is due to the osmotic effect of glucose alone.

Hyponatremia in this situation is described as translocational hyponatremia

Management should be control of diabetes mellitus and not administration of Na containing fluid.

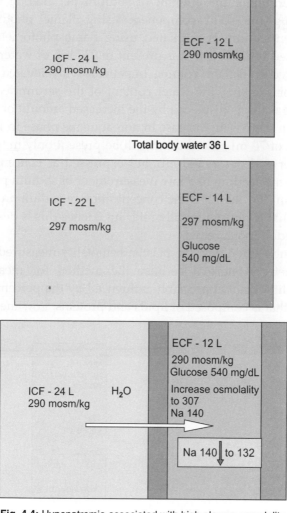

Fig. 4.4: Hyponatremia associated with high plasma osmolality

Isotonic Hyponatremia (Pseudohyponatremia)

Plasma volume is normally constituted by of 930 mL of water and 70 mL of non-aqueous solutes like proteins and lipids. Most of the clinical laboratories measure sodium concentration by determining the amount of sodium per liter of serum, including the solid component using flame photometer. So when sodium is estimated using flame photometer, the measured sodium is that is present in 930 mL of water but is expressed in 1000 mL volume. In patients with elevated serum lipids or proteins, the water content of the serum decreases because water is displaced by the increased amount of solids. So when there is an increase in non-aqueous phase to 100 mL instead of 70 mL, the sodium will be present only in 900 mL of water and not in 930 mL, but expressed as concentration in 1000 mL leading to a low measurement of sodium per liter of serum (Fig. 4.5). It is the concentration of sodium in serum water that is physiologically relevant. Hence this is described as Pseudohyponatremia.

In such situations, the plasma osmolality measured using osmometer is normal because the method for measuring osmolality is not appreciably influenced by the percentage of serum that is composed of lipids and proteins. Low measured

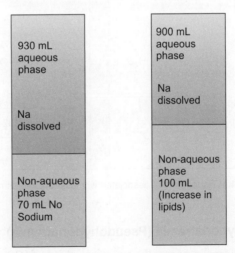

140 / 930 x 1000 = 151 meq /L   151 / 900 x 1000 = 135.9 meq / L

Fig. 4.5: Changes in ECF sodium with increase in non-aqueous phase due to lipids/proteins

plasma sodium give a low calculated plasma osmolality. Since measured osmolality is normal, there will be an osmolar gap. Pseudohyponatremia is diagnosed if hyponatremia is associated with a normal measured plasma osmolality despite hyponatremia. Causes of pseudohyponatremia are hyperglobulinemias and hypertriglyceridemia. These conditions are very rare. This can be overcome by the use of ion selective electrodes.

Correction Factor for Increased Proteins

Decrease in plasma Na in millimol/L
= {Plasma protein level [in grams per deciliter] – 8} × 0.25

When proteins increase by 4g, Na will decrease only by 1 mmol/L. For a significant reduction in Na value, proteins have to be very high. This is very rarely encounterd in clinical situations.

Case History 3

A patient with Waldenstroms Macroglobulinemia on routine lab evaluation had Na of 134 mmol/L. He was asymptomatic and was euvolemic.

Laboratory parameters are as follows:

Parameter	value
RBS	126 mg%
Urea	20 mg%
Sodium	134 mmol/L
Potassium	4 mmol/L
Serum proteins	12 g%

Step 1: To calculate osmolality. The osmolality is 286 mosmoles/kg. Hence, this is isoosmolar hyponatremia.
Step 2: Correction factor for increased proteins
{Plasma protein level [in grams per deciliter] – 8} × 0.25 =
decrease in plasma Na (in millimoles/L) (12 – 8) × 0.25 =
1 mmol/L. In this patient Na is only 134, just outside normal. This is Isotonic hyponatremia (Pseudohyponatremia)

Correction Factor for Increased Lipids

Decrease in plasma Na level (in millimoles/ L) = Triglyceride level (in milligrams per deciliter) × 0.002

For the Na to decrease by 1 mmol/L, Triglcerides level should be 500 mg% This is of theoretical interest only.

Hypoosmolar (Hypotonic) Hyponatremia

Why Recognize Hyponatremia?

Acute onset of hyponatremia is important clinically because:

1. Acute severe hyponatremia can cause substantial morbidity and mortality due to neurological complications.
2. Hyponatremia, has been shown to contribute to a high mortality in patients with coronary artery disease, cirrhosis liver with ascites, and other underlying diseases and
3. Rapid correction of chronic hyponatremia can cause severe neurologic deficits-osmotic demyelination syndrome and death.

Most patients with chronic hyponatremia are asymptomatic and hyponatremia should not be aggressively corrected.

Pathophysiology

When there is a sodium deficit and hypotonicity, whatever may be the cause, certain physiological adaptations occur. Sodium is not freely permeable, hence water shifts to the cells to achieve osmotic equilibrium. This will cause cerebral edema. The adaptive mechanisms for correction of hyponatremia take several days. Hence, acute hyponatremia is symptomatic and has to be corrected appropriately.

The consequences are seen mainly in the brain. Brain volume is usually regulated by equalization of ECF and ICF osmolality. Hyponatremia and resulting reduced osmolality leads to an influx of water into the brain, primarily through glial cells and largely via the water channel aquaporin (AQP). Water is then shunted to astrocytes which swell, largely preserving the neurons.

On the other hand, if hyponatremia is persistent for more than 48 hours, adaptations to the hypoosmolar condition occur. Adaptive mechanisms in hyponatremia are mediated through

- Na-K ATPase system,
- Aquaporin channels, and
- Organic osmolytes.

Na is extruded at the same time using Na-K ATPase system. Potassium extrusion follow Na, but is slower.

It has been shown that inorganic osmolytes and organic osmolytes (e.g. glycine, taurine, creatine and myoinositol) move from cells during hypoosmolar states.

If hyponatremia is corrected to normal or hypertonic state, the reverse happens. Cells will get dehydrated due to rapid shift of water from the cells. Previously, this pathological injury was described only in the pons, hence, it was described as central pontine myelinolysis (CPM). Now it has been shown that other parts of brain are also affected and is now described as osmotic demyelination syndrome (ODS).

CLINICAL FEATURES OF HYPONATREMIA

Hyponatremia is reported in 20 to 45% of sick hospitalized children. Incidence of hyponatremia is higher during the peak southwest monsoon season. Humidity and temperature may have important role in the manifestations of hyponatremia. Symptoms depend on

- Age of the patient,
- Rate of fall in sodium,
- Whether it is acute or chronic (Acute—if the problem developed within 48 hours and chronic if there is no documented normal Na value within 48 hours).

Patients can present with:

- Symptoms of associated disease—heart failure, cirrhosis liver, chronic kidney disease.
- Neurological symptoms causd by hyponatremia.
- Those that arise from rapid overcorrection

• Detected during routine biochemical work up and may be totally asymptomatic.

Hyponatremic Encephalopathy

Symptoms can be due to neurological involvement—can range from malaise, nausea to alteration of sensorium and seizures. As mentioned earlier decrease in osmolality can result in brain edema. Skull can accommodate only upto 10% increase in volume. If increase in volume is very rapid and more than 10%, brain herniation and death may ensue.

Hypotonic Hyponatremia (True Hyponatremia)

True hyponatremia as has been emphasized is always hypoosmolar. This is almost always due to inability of the kidney to increase free water clearance.

This is classified based on fluid status into hypovolemic, euvolemic and hypervolemic hyponatremia (Fig. 4.6).

Hypotonic Hyponatremia

The following steps are used to evaluate hypotonic hyponatremia:

Step 1: Calculate the plasma osmolality
Step 2: Clinical assessment of ECF volume
Step 3: Estimate urine sodium

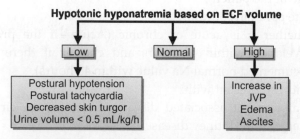

Fig. 4.6: Hypotonic hyponatremia based on ECF volume

Step 4: Estimate urine potassium to find out the cause of increased Na loss in urine.

Step 1: Calculate the plasma osmolality. If the osmolality is low, it is true hyponatremia.

Step 2: Clinical assessment of ECF volume — Since the ECF volume cannot be directly measured, this is assessed clinically (Fig. 4.6). *Bedside signs of hypovolemia:*

- Early signs of hypovolemia are postural hypotension and Postural tachycardia.
- Persistent hypotension and tachycardia indicate moderate reduction in ECF volume.
- Diminished skin turgor is best elicited on the anterior abdominal wall.
- Increased longitudinal furrowing of tongue is another sign.
- Urine volume < 500 mL in 24 hours or 0.5 mL/kg per hour.

Step 3: Estimate urine sodium — (refer Fig. 4.7) sodium loss can occur through renal or extra renal route. In Hypovolemic hyponatremia, to find out the route of loss of Na whether renal or extrarenal, estimate urine sodium. If urine *sodium is less than 10 mmol/L it is due to extrarenal cause and if more than 20 mmol/L it is due to renal loss.*

Step 4: To find out the cause of renal Na loss, estimate urine potassium (refer Fig. 4.8) — If urine potassium is more than 20 mmol/L, it can be due to tubular wasting of Na and K either due to interstitial disease or diuretic use. Vomiting can also result in high urine K.

High urine Na and low urine K is suggestive of diminished adrenal response.

Case History 4

A 50-year-old woman was admitted with alteration of sensorium. Past history included hypertension and she was on hydrochlorthiazide treatment. Systemic history was unremarkable. Metalazone was added for releiving edema as on examination her BP was 110/70 mm Hg in the supine position and 90/60 mm Hg in sitting posture. Pulse rate was 110/min and had diminished skin turgor. Her weight is 60 kg. Her urine volume was 200 mL in last 24 hours.

Laboratory parameters are as follows:

Parameter	Value
RBS	90 mg%
Serum creatinine	1.2 mg%
Urea	60 mg%
Sodium	118 mmol/L
Potassium	3.1 mmol/L

Step 1: Find out the osmolality

$$P_{osm} = \frac{90 \text{ mg/dL} + 60 \text{ mg/dL}}{18} + \frac{2 \,[122 \text{ mmol/L}) + 3.1 \text{ mmol/L}]}{6}$$

= 265 milliosmoles/kg

she has hypotonic hyponatremia.

Step 2: Assess ECF volume—This lady has clinical signs of ECF volume depletion as she had postural hypotension, tachycardia, diminished skin turgor and is oliguric.

Step 3: Estimate urine sodium

Parameter	Value
Urine sodium	30 millimoles/L
Urine potassium	33 millmoles/L

In this patient urine sodium was 30 mmol/L and indicates renal loss of Na.

Step 4: Estimate urine potassium—Urine potassium was 35 mmol/L suggesting diuretics as the cause of hypovolemic hyponatremia.

She was managed with withdrawal of diuretics and sodium supplements

Final diagnosis: This elderly lady had hypovolemic hyponatremia, increased sodium and potassium loss in urine. Metalazone which was added to thiazides for treatment of her edema had precipitated hyponatremia

Causes of hyponatremia due to increased sodium loss in urine, and causes for extra renal loss of sodium is shown in Figure 4.7.

Step 4: To find out the etiology of renal Na loss, estimate urine potassium. If urinary K loss is less than 20 millimoles/L, hypoaldosteronism should be suspected (Fig. 4.8).

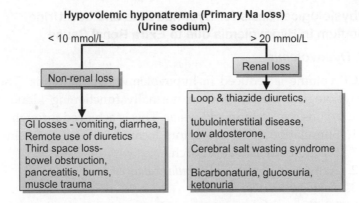

Fig. 4.7: Hypovolemic hyponatremia—Causes based on urine sodium loss

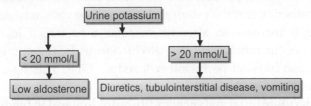

Fig. 4.8: Hypovolemic hyponatremia—Causes based on urine potassium loss

Rationale for Estimating Urine Sodium to Find out the Cause of Sodium Loss

In a hypovolemic patient, GFR will be low and the physiological mechanisms of glomerulotubular balance and tubuloglomerular feedback will be activated. Renal tubules will avidly reabsorb sodium and can result in low urinary sodium. This indicates normal kidney function and the cause is extrarenal for Na loss.

In hypovolemic patient, failure to conserve sodium by the tubules resulting in sodium loss in urine can be due to:

- Loop and thiazide diuretics
- Diseases of tubulointerstitium
- Low aldosterone.

Physiological Basis for Hyponatremia and Low Urine Sodium in Hypovolemia due to Extra Renal Cause

1. Hypovolemia

ECF volume is reduced in hypovolemic hyponatremia. The physiological mechanisms in normally functioning kidneys are to conserve sodium and water. This is achieved through

1. Stimulation of baroreceptors located in the great veins, carotid body and aortic arch.
2. Activation of *glomerulotubular balance.*
3. *Tubuloglomerular feedback.*

Stimulation of baroreceptors — Hypovolemia stimulates the baroreceptors located in the great veins, carotid body and aortic arch. There is decrease in stretch. This will stimulate the sympathetic nervous system and there will be vasoconstriction. There is increase in afferent vascular tone which leads to reduction in renal perfusion. Reduction in ECF volume and reduction in renal perfusion will reduce GFR. This results in reduced excretion of sodium in urine.

Glomerulotubular balance and tubuloglomerular feedback: When there is low GFR, glomerulotubular feedback is activated and there will be increased in proximal tubular reabsorption of solutes and water.

This increased reabsorption will reduce the delivery to the distal tubule. This will stimulate of Renin Angiotensin Aldosterone System (RAAS). There is increased reabsorption of sodium (chapter 3.8, Fig. 3.2). This will reduce the delivery of water to the diluting segments of the nephron. Thus, free water excretion will be decreased. Low urine sodium in presence of hyponatremia suggest an extra renal cause for loss of sodium.

2. Hypoosmolality

Low osmolality stimulates thirst and there will be increase in water intake. Decreased free water excretion coupled with increase in fluid intake produce hyponatremia

Causes of Hypovolemic Hyponatremia

- Blood loss, Plasma loss as in burns,
- Third space loss (bowel obstruction, pancreatitis),
- GI losses-diarrhea, vomiting

Vomiting: Gastric juice contains chloride more than sodium. In vomiting the metabolic abnormalities are due to ECF volume contraction and renal compensatory mechanisms. This results in hyponatremic, hypokalemic metabolic alkalosis (Fig. 4.9).

Management will consist of correction of ECF volume contraction with isotonic saline and hypokalemia with potassium supplements.

Diarrhea: Diarrhea is associated with loss of potassium and bicarbonate in stools. This will cause hyponatremic, hypokalemic metabolic acidosis. Correction of hyponatremia and hypokalemia is by infusion of Ringer's lactate and isotonic saline. Bicarbonate infusion may be given if pH is less than 7.1.

Specific therapy for the underlying disorder should be initiated; antiemetics and antidiarrheal agents can be used as appropriate. Hypertonic saline is not required since these patients are volume depleted also.

Management of Hypovolemic Hyponatremia

1. Withdrawal of cause, if possible and correction of underlying disorder.

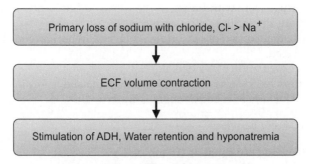

Fig. 4.9: Sequence of events in vomiting

2. Look for clinical signs of hypovolemia.
3. In life threatening situations, isotonic saline is to be started and hemodynamic stability should be attained.
4. When hypovolemia is doubtful, fluid challenge with isotonic saline 500–1000 mL can be tried.

Indication for Correction of Sodium Deficit

1. Symptomatic hyponatremia.
2. Acute hyponatremia (Na < 110 mmol/L).

Treatment Guidelines for Saline Administration

Rate of infusion should be
- 0.5 mmol/L/h in mild to moderate hyponatremia
- 2–3 mmol/L/h in the first 2 to 3 hours in patients with seizures
- Permissible total correction is 8 mmol/L in 8 hours and maximum rise of 10 to 12 mmol/L in 24 hours

Calculation of Sodium Deficit

Sodium deficit can be calculated using the Formula:
Total body water × (Normal Na-patient's Na)

Management of Case History 4

Step 1: Withdrawal of the offending agent.
She had received thiazides with recent addition of metalazone. These drugs were withdrawn.
Is there any indication for correction?
She had alteration of sensorium and hence hypornatremia has to be corrected.
Step 2: Calculation of Na deficit
Sodium deficit was calculated based on the above formula.
In 60 kg lady 55% body weight is water

Total body water = $\dfrac{55 \times 60}{100}$ = 33 L

Patient had a sodium of 118 mmol/L
Na deficit = 33 × (140 – 118) = 726 mmol.

ECF volume is low and aim is to correct the deficit with normal saline. 1 liter of normal saline contains 154 millimoles of sodium chloride.

Hence, volume of normal saline required in liters to raise Na from 118 to 126 (the permissible daily rise in Na in 24 hours is 8 mmol.) (60 Kg × 55%) × (126 – 118) = 33 × 8 = 264 mmol.

Step 3: Calculate the volume of normal saline required?

1 liter of normal saline contains 154 mmoles of Na, to give 264 mmoles the volume of normal saline required is 264 ÷ 154 = 1.7 liters. As mentioned earlier guidelines had to be strictly followed for correction of hyponatremia.

Formula 2 is used to find out rate of rise in sodium with infusion of sodium containing fluids.

Rate of rise of Na in mmol/L = Na in infusate-patient's Na/(TBW + 1)

If Potassium containing fluids are used

(Na + K) in infusate - patient's Na/(TBW + 1)

Step 4: To find out the rate of rise in sodium with infusion of one liter of normal saline. Formula 2 is applied

So in the above patient rate of rise of Na in mmol/L with infusion of one liter of normal saline

= 154 – 118/(33 + 1) = 36/34 = 1.05 mmol

The permissible rise in Na is 0.5 to 1 mmol/L/h,

Hence, this patient can receive 500 mL to 1000 mL/h.

During infusion serum sodium was checked fourth hourly. Saline infusion was stopped when her sensorium became normal and sodium reached 125 mmol/L.

In symptomatic hyponatremia, hypertonic saline can be used but extreme caution should be taken to see that the rate of increase does not exceed 5–8 mmol/L/day. Recurrence of hyponatremia is high with thiazides and so should not be challenged with thiazides again. If diuretic therapy is essential in such a patient, the serum [Na] should be measured within a few days after initiation of treatment and frequently with in the first several weeks.

Causes of Hypovolemic Hyponatremia with High Sodium in Urine

- Loop and thiazide diuretics
- Diseases of tubulointerstitium,
- Low aldosterone

Case History 5

A 20-year-old male is admitted with diarrhea and altered sensorium. Past history is unremarkable. On examination patient is drowsy, BP 80/60 mm Hg, heart rate 110/min, CVP 4 mm Hg.

Laboratory parameters are as follows

Parameter	Value
RBS	108 mg%
Urea	60 mg%
Sodium	115 mmol/L
Potassium	3 mmol/L
Plasma osmolality	246 milliosmoles (2x Na)

Step 1: Find out the osmolality
P_{osm} = 108mg/18 + 60/6 + 2 × (115)
    = 246 milliosmoles/kg
He has hypotonic hyponatremia.
Step 2: This gentle man has clinical signs of ECF volume depletion as he had postural hypotension, tachycardia, and CVP of 4 mm of Hg.
Step 3: Estimate urine sodium

Parameter	Value
Urine sodium	5 millimoles/L
Urine potassium	10 millmoles/L

In this patient urine sodium is 5 mmol/L and indicates extra renal loss of Na.
Step 4: Urine potassium is 10 mmol/L suggesting diarrhea as the cause of hypokalemia with hypovolemic hyponatremia.

This 20-year-old male has hypovolemic hyponatremia, decreased sodium and potassium in urine. The cause of Na loss is due to diarrhea as indicated by low urine Na and urine K.

Hyponatremia with Expanded ECF Volume

ECF volume expansion can be due to administration of hypotonic fluids, effect of ADH, fluid retention due to acute kidney injury (AKI) or chronic kidney disease (CKD). Drugs mainly diuretics and diseases of the renal interstitium can affect urinary dilution. Failure to generate solute free dilute urine can also result in hyponatremia.

Clinical Features of ECF Volume Expansion

Patients may have raised JVP, edema and ascites.

Hyponatremia with Low Effective Arterial Blood Volume (EABV) Effective Arterial Blood Volume

Collection of large volumes of fluid can occur in serous cavities due to leakage from the capillaries. This can cause low EABV *but the total ECF volume will be normal.* Hence, weight of the patient will not increase.

Common conditions associated with third space loss are ascites, cellulitis, pleural effusion, paralytic ileus, etc. (Fig. 4.10). Though the total volume remains unchanged, the effective arterial blood volume is low. Low effective arterial blood volume (EABV) will stimulate ADH, leading to water retention and further dilution.

When the effective arterial blood volume (EABV) is low, there will be conservation of Na and H_2O and urine sodium will be low. In AKI and CKD the decrease in GFR is due to intrinsic renal disease and renal response is altered. Hence, excretion of sodium in urine will be high.

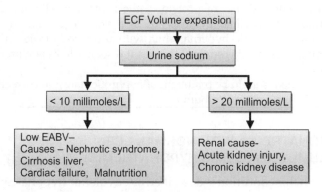

Fig. 4.10: Causes of hyponatremia with ECF volume expansion based on urine sodium loss

Case History 6

A 15-year-old adolescent male gives history of nephrotic syndrome. He had normal blood pressure, normal GFR, and no other comorbid factors. On examination he has raised JVP, is edematous, has ascites. Systemic examination is unremarkable. Laboratory parameters are as follows

Blood Parameter	Value
RBS	90 mg%
Creatinine	1 mg%
Urea	20 mg%
Na	126 mmol/L
K	4 mmol/L
Plasma osmolality	268 mosmoles
Serum albumin	2.5 gm/dL

Step 1: Find out the osmolality
P_{osm} = 90 mg/dL/18 + 20 mg/dL/6 + 2 × (126 + 4)
     = 268 milliosmoles/kg
Patient has hypotonic hyponatremia.
Step 2: Assess ECF Volume—
    This gentleman has clinical signs of ECF volume expansion as he has ascites and edema.
Step 3 Estimate urine sodium

Parameter	Value
Urine Sodium	6 millimoles/L

This patient had loss of protein in the urine, low albumin and normal GFR. He had evidence of ECF volume expansion. He also had hypotonic hypernatremia with urine sodium less than 10 millimoles/L. This suggest that renal response to hyponatremia is normal.
Management should be treatment of nephrotic state and correction of EABV with plasma/albumin

HYPONATREMIA WITH NORMAL ECF VOLUME (EUVOLEMIC HYPONATREMIA)

Though this condition is described as euvolemic hyponatremia, there is excess of total body water. They have no signs of fluid expansion because the fluid is retained inside the cells. Sodium is diluted in excess of body water resulting in hyponatremia. This is because of

1. State of inappropriate ADH secretion
2. An inappropriate sensitivity of the kidney tubules to vasopressin,
3. Impaired free water clearance with or without excessive water intake.

Syndrome of Inappropriate ADH Secretion (SIADH)

SIADH (which is now also known as SIAD-syndrome of inappropriate diuresis) is characterized by euvolumic hyponatremia.

Pathophysiology

Physiological stimuli for ADH secretion are hypovolemia and hyperosmolality. When there is low ECF volume or high plasma osmolality, Posterior pituitary secretes ADH and collecting duct responds to ADH by insertion of water channels – aquaporins. Water will be shifted from tubular lumen to systemic circulation. This will correct low ECF volume and osmolality. This will result in concentrated urine and urine Na will be more than 40 mmol/L. In physiological circumstances plasma osmolality will be high and urine osmolality will be appropriately high.

In SIADH, ADH secretion is not in response to high osmolality or low ECF volume. In spite of normal plasma volume and plasma osmolality, ADH is secreted from the normal site or from an ectopic site. Increased secretion of ADH without an appropriate stimulus of hypovolemia or hyperosmolality will impair free water clearance and result in water retention. This will dilute the sodium and result in hyponatremia. This is called SIADH.

Inappropriate Release of ADH from Normal Site

Common causes are:

1. Tumor, trauma, infection, cerebrovascular accident, subarachnoid hemorrhage, Guillain-Barré syndrome, delirium tremens, multiple sclerosis.
2. Surgery – Postoperative
3. AIDS
4. Prolonged strenuous exercise (marathon, triathlon, ultramarathon, hot-weather hiking)
5. Potomania
6. Drugs—Exogenous vasopressin, nonsteroidal antiinflammatory drugs, ncotine, diuretics, chlorpropamide, carbamazepine, tricyclic antidepressants, SSRIs, vincristine, thioridazine, cyclophosphamide, clofibrate, bomocriptine, haloperidol, thiothixene, exogenous oxytocin, MAOIs.
7. Idiopathic.

ADH from an Ectopic Site

Causes are:

1. Pulmonary disease—Tumor, pneumonia, chronic obstructive pulmonary disease, lung abscess, tuberculosis, cystic fibrosis.
2. Carcinoma—Lung, pancreas, thymus, ovary, lymphoma.
3. Positive pressure ventilation.

CRITERIA TO DIAGNOSE SIADH (BARTTER AND SCHWARTZ)

- Plasma osmolality < 275 mosm/kg
- Urine osmolality > 100 mosm/kg with normal renal function
- Euvolumia—absence of signs of hypovolemia or ECF volume expansion, edema or ascites
- Urine Na > 40 mmol/L
  and is associated with low urea, creatinine and uric acid due to dilution.

Other causes of ADH release should be excluded
• Hypothyroidism
• Hypocortisolism
• Chronic liver disease.

Classification of causes of euvolemic hyponatremia based on urine osmolality and Na loss in urine is shown in Figure 4.11.

Case History 7

A 30-year-old gentleman with no premorbid illness was admitted with vomiting and diagnosed to have aseptic meningitis. He had no history of any drug intake. There was no h/o any significant past illness. On examination he is drowsy, hypovolemic. His weight is 70 kg. His blood pressure is 90/60 mm Hg and has tachycardia. Laboratory parameters are as follows:

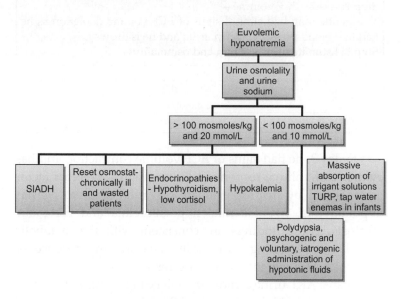

Fig. 4.11: Approach to euvolemic hyponatremia

Parameter	Day 3	Day 5
Urinalysis	normal	normal
Plasma glucose	108 mg%	90 mg%
Plasma urea	60 mg%	15 mg%
Plasma creatinine	1.2 mg%	0.6 mg%
Serum Na	130 mmol/L	117mmol /L
Serum K	3 mmol/L	4 mmol/L
Bicarbonate	32 mmol/L	24 mmol/L
Chloride	84 mmol/L	82 mmol/L
Plasma osmolality	282 mosm/kg	249 mosm/kg

Analysis of Day 3 Investigations

Step 1: Find out the osmolality
P_{osm} = 108 mg/18 + 60/6 + 2 (130 + 3)
= 282 milliosmoles/kg
Patient has hypotonic hyponatremia.

Step 2: Assess ECF volume—
This gentle man had clinical signs of ECF volume depletion as he had low blood pressure, tachycardia and he is drowsy.

Step 3: Estimate urine sodium and osmolality

Parameter	Value
Urine sodium	60 mmol/L
Chloride	6 mmol/L
Osmolality	450 mosm/kg

On day 3, he had signs of ECF volume contraction and has evidence of volume responsive kidney injury. Prerenal factor is suggested by disproportionate elevation of urea. He has hyponatremia, hypokalemia, hypochloremia and metabolic alkalosis. These findings are consistent with the metabolic sequelae of vomiting. Low urine chloride in presence of hypochloremia suggests adequate renal response. In volume responsive AKI, urine osmolality will be high. This patient also had a relatively high urine osmolality. *Volume responsive AKI usually has a low urine sodium concentration* but this patient had high sodium loss and low urine chloride. High urine sodium in this patient may be due to the excretion of sodium with another anion $HCO3^-$ He was managed with normal saline and other supportive measures.

Analysis of Day 5 Investigations

Step 1: Find out the osmolality

P_{osm} = 90 mg/18 + 15/6 + 2 (117 + 4)

    = 249 milliosmoles/kg

Patient had hypotonic hyponatremia.

Step 2: Assess ECF volume—

    This gentleman has no clinical signs of ECF volume depletion or volume expansion

Step 3: Estimate urine sodium and osmolality

Parameter	Value
Urine sodium	50 mosm/L
Chloride	48 mosm/L
Osmolality	407 mosm/kg

On day 5, he was euvolumic. His GFR was normal, sodium decreased further, hypochloremia persisted, bicarbonate normalized. Urine electrolytes showed increased loss of sodium and chloride with osmolality of 407 mosmoles/kg.

He was diagnosed to have euvolumic hyponatremia with hyperosmolar urine and increased sodium loss in urine.

He had no premorbid illness, thyroid and adrenal functions were normal. Potassium was normal. Hence, probable cause is syndrome of inappropriate anti-diuretic hormone (SIADH) due to aseptic meningitis.

Management of SIADH

The single most important factor guiding initial therapy is the presence of neurologic symptoms.

Acute hyponatremia is arbitrarily defined as hyponatremia < 48 hours duration and are usually symptomatic

If the hyponatremia is severe < 120 mmol/L and/or there is high risk for neurologic complications, hyponatremia should be corrected to higher serum [Na$^+$] levels promptly.

Patients with more chronic hyponatremia (>48 hours duration) have minimal neurologic symptoms and are at little risk from complications of hyponatremia. These patients can develop osmotic demyelination following rapid correction.

Management of SIADH (SIAD) Consists of

1. Identifying the cause of SIADH.
2. Fluid restriction
3. Saline administration
4. Pharmacologic therapy.

1. Identifying the Cause of SIADH

If a primary cause like tumor is identified, resection of the tumor corrects hyponatremia. If infection is the cause, treatment of infection will help to correct hyponatremia.

2. Fluid Restriction

Water retention is responsible for low Na in hypervolumic and euvolumic hyponatremia. Hence *fluid restriction* is the mainstay of therapy. Points to be remembered are:

1. All fluids, not only water, must be included in the restriction.
2. The degree of restriction required depends on urine output plus insensible fluid loss -that is nonsolid food fluids should be limited to 500 mL/day below the average daily urine volume.
3. Several days of restriction are usually necessary before a significant increase in plasma osmolality occurs. Only fluid should be restricted. Na intake should not be restricted. Because the loss of sodium in urine continues, a relatively high intake of NaCl is to be given.
4. Small dose of loop diuretic is useful when there is associated cardiovascular disease.

3. Saline Administration

If hyponatremia is severe and associated with neurological manifestations, hypertonic (3%) saline is used. Sodium deficit, volume of fluid required, and rate of rise in Na are found out by using the formulae and steps are as shown earlier for hypovolemic hyponatremia.

The approximate infusion rate of 3% saline / hour =

weight in kg × required rate of rise of sodium

Example: In 60 kg man, if the required rise is 1 mmol/L/h, the rate of infusion of 3% saline is 60 × 1 = 60 mL/h If the required rise is 0.5 mmol/L/h, the rate of infusion should be 30 mL/h.

Indications for Interruption of Acute Treatment

End points are:

1. The patient's symptoms are abolished;
2. A safe serum [Na$^+$] level (generally > 120 mmol/L) is achieved; or
3. A total magnitude of correction of 8 mmol/L is achieved, serum sodium should be monitored every 2 hours or at least once in 4 hours.

    Sodium should be corrected to safe limits and not to normal levels.

    Na concentrations of hypertonic sodium containing fluids used in practice are shown below.

- 5% NaCl in water – 855 mmol/L
- 3% NaCl in water – 513 mmol/L

4. Pharmacologic Therapy of SIADH

Indications

- If hyponatremia does not resolve with fluid restriction
- If urine osmolality is very high and patient cannot tolerate severe restriction,

    Drugs used are demeclocycline, urea and vasopressin receptor antagonists vaptans.

Demeclocycline

This agent causes a nephrogenic form of diabetes insipidus, thereby decreasing urine concentration even in the presence of high plasma AVP levels. Appropriate doses of demeclocycline range from 600 to 1,200 mg/day administered in divided doses. Treatment must be continued for several days to achieve maximal diuretic effects. Consequently one should wait for 3 to 4 days before deciding to increase the dose.

Disadvantages—Cause reversible azotemia and sometimes nephrotoxicity, especially in patients with cirrhosis. Renal function should therefore be monitored in patients treated with demeclocycline on a regular basis, and the medication should be discontinued if increasing azotemia is noted.

Urea

Produces osmotic diuresis. Dose is 30 g/day.

Disadvantages—Tablet form is not available,unpalatable taste and in very high doses can precipitate severe azotemia.

Agonists selective for ê-opioid receptors

Clinical trials have successfully produced aquaresis in patients with cirrhosis.

Vasopressin Receptor Antagonists or Vaptans

Conivaptan is FDA approved drug for clinical use in euvolemic and hypervolemic hyponatremia in hospitalized patients, *not used in patients with congestive heart failure (CHF) or cirrhosis.*

Mechanism of action—Blocks the binding of vasopressin to the receptors in the distal nephron and inhibits the insertion of aquaporin-2 channels into the membrane. This results in increased free water clearance and increase serum sodium concentration.

Dose and route of administration—A bolus of 20 mg over 30 minutes in 100 mL of 5% dextrose is given intravenously followed by infusion of 20 mg in 100 mL of 5% dextrose over 24 hours. Sodium is monitored every 2 to 4 hours, and the dose may be titrated to 40 mg per 24 hours to obtain an increase in sodium of 0.5 to 1.0 mmol/L per hour. Fluid is restricted to 1.5 to 2 liters per day.

Tolvaptan -available as 15mg and 30 mg tablets - oral preparation. indications and contra indications same as for Conivaptan. Guidelines for correction of hyponatremia are the same as for hypovolemic hyponatremia.

Relative contraindications — Renal disease, hepatic impairment, cardiac failure.

Caution — Avoid inhibitors of the cytochrome P-450 3A4 isoenzyme (CYP3A4) including ketoconazole, itraconazole, clarithromycin, ritanavir, and indinavir.

Osmotic Demyelination Syndrome which is seen with rapid correction of hyponatremia is not described with Vaptan therapy

---

Reviewing the case history, his weight is 70 kg, plasma Na is 117 mmol/L

Step 1: Treat the cause

Since, no specific treatment is available for aseptic meningitis patient was managed symptomatically

Step 2: Fluid restriction

Since, his urine volume was 1000 mL, nonsolid fluid intake was restricted to 500 mL.

Step 3: Saline administration

To find out the volume of saline required, sodium deficit was calculated based on the first formula.

In 70 kg young man 60% of body weight is water. patient had a sodium of 117 mmol/L

Na deficit = (70 Kg × 60%) × (140–117) = 42 × 23 = 966 mmol.

ECF volume is normal and aim is to correct the deficit with hypertonic saline.

Volume of hypertonic saline required in liters to raise Na to normal value

= 966 ÷ 513 = 1.88 Liters

In this patient, since the permissible daily rise in Na is only 8 mmol/L in 24 hours, initial correction should be to 126 mmol/L.

Na deficit = (70 Kg × 60%) × (126 – 117) = 42 × 9 = 378 mmol.

Volume of hypertonic saline required is calculated as follows:

1 liter of hypertonic saline contains 513 mmols of Na, to give 378 mmoles the volume of hypertonic saline required is 378 ÷ 513 = 730 mL.

to find out the rate of rise in sodium with infusion of 1 liter of hypertonic saline

Rate of rise of Na in mmol/L = 513 – 117 ÷ (42 + 1) = 396/43 = 9.2 mmol

As the total permissible rise in 24 hr is 8 to 12 mmol and permissible rise in hour is 0.5 to 1 mmol/L, patient can receive 700 mL in 24 hours.

During infusion serum sodium was checked fourth hourly. Saline infusion was stopped when her sensorium became normal and sodium reached 125 mmol/L.

Case History 8

A 50-year-old lady is admitted with history headache and generalized seizures. Systemic history was negative for hypertension, seizure disorder or any other disease. The only past history was chronic headache which was managed as migraine. On examination she was drowsy, vital signs were normal, euvolemic, BP was 110/70 mm Hg, optic fundi were normal. There was no focal neurological deficit

Laboratory Parameters are as follows:

Parameter	Value
RBS	110 mg%
Urea	11 mg%
Creatinine	0.4 mg%
Uric acid	
Na	106 mmol/L
K	4.4 mmol/L
Plasma osmolality	228 mosm/Kg

Step 1: Find out the osmolality

P_{osm} = 110 mg/dL/18 + 11 mg/dL/6 + 2 × (106 + 4.4)
   = 228 milliosmoles/kg

Patient has hypotonic hyponatremia.

Step 2: Assess ECF volume

This lady has no clinical signs of ECF volume depletion or volume expansion and was euvolumic

Step 3: Estimate urine sodium and osmolality

Parameter	Value
Urine sodium	60 mosm/L
Osmolality	423 mosm/kg

This patient had severe hypotonic hyponatremia with inappropriately high urine osmolality to plasma osmolality and increased loss of sodium in urine. Urea and uric acid were low suggesting dilution. Patient had no other comorbid conditions.

She had no hypotension or clinical signs to suggest hypothyroidism, adrenal disease, liver disease or cardiac failure.

Step 1: Treat the cause

Her seizures were controlled with anti-convulsants.

Step 2: Fluid restriction

She was managed with nonfood fluids of 800 mL/day, since her urine volume was only 1400 mL.

Step 3: Saline administration

To find out the volume of saline required, sodium deficit was calculated based on the first formula.

In 43 kg lady, 55% body weight is water. Patient had a sodium of 117mmol/L

Na deficit = (43 × 55/100) × (140 – 106) = 34 × 23.65
= 804 mmol.

ECF volume is normal and aim is to correct the deficit with hypertonic saline.

Volume of hypertonic saline required in liters to raise Na to normal value = 804 ÷ 513 = 1.57 Liters

In this patient, since the permissible rise in Na in 24 hours is only 8 mmol/L, initial correction should be to 114mmol/L.

Na deficit = (43 Kg × 55%) × (114 – 106) = 189 mmol.

Volume of hypertonic saline required was calculated as follows

One liter of hypertonic saline contains 513 mmols of Na, to give 368 mmoles the volume of hypertonic saline required is 189 ÷ 513 = 368 mL

To find out the rate of rise in sodium with infusion of 1 liter of hypertonic saline

Rate of rise of Na in mmol/L = 513 – 106 ÷ (23.65 + 1)
= 16 mmol/L

This patient can receive 500 mL in 24 hours.

During infusion serum sodium was checked fourth hourly. Saline infusion was stopped when her sensorium became normal and sodium reached 114 mmol/L.

To exclude endocrine conditions, T_3, T_4, TSH and plasma cortisol were sent.

Hormone	Value
T_3	60
T_4	2
TSH	2.4 (0.34–4.25 mIU/L)
Fasting plasma cortisol	< 1 μg/dL

This was suggestive of central hypothyroidism and hypo-adrenalism. MRI brain showed empty sella syndrome. Patient was started on prednisolone 7.5 mg and 100 μg of thyroxine

There is no recurrence of hyponatremia and patient is on regular follow up

HYPONATREMIA IN SPECIAL SITUATIONS

- Neurological disorders
- Post-TURP syndrome
- Primary polydipsia
- Exercise-associated hyponatremia (EAH)
- In neonates and children
- Beer potomania.

Neurological Disorders

This is a commonly encountered electrolyte abnormality in patients with neurological disorders. This can contribute to worsening of neurological status. Prompt identification and judicious correction as mentioned earlier can reverse the problem.

There are three important causes for hyponatremia:

- Syndrome of inappropriate antidiuretic hormone (SIADH)
- Cerebral salt wasting syndrome (CSWS)
- Nephrogenic syndrome of inappropriate antidiuresis
  SIADH is discussed earlier in this chapter.

Cerebral Salt Wasting Syndrome (CSWS)

Peters et al described this condition in 1950. There is a renal sodium transport abnormality in patients with intracranial disease. This leads to the development of extracellular volume depletion. As in SIADH, thyroid and adrenal function will be normal. Since, hyponatremia is due to renal Na wasting, more appropriate term will be renal salt wasting syndrome [RSW]. Pathogenesis is not definitely known.

Factors implicated are

1. Derangements of sympathetic nervous system
2. Stimulation of kidneys
3. Production of digoxin-like peptides,
4. Excess natriuretic factors

With interruption to sympathetic inputs, there is decreased renal sodium reabsorption in the proximal nephron. This ultimately leads to a large delivery of sodium to the distal nephron, increased sodium excretion, and a decrease in EABV. The decrease in EABV in turn activates baroreceptor stimulated AVP release.

Another proposed mechanism is excessive central release of one or more natriuretic factors such as atrial natriuretic peptide (ANP) or brain natriuretic peptide (BNP). Both these factors increase urinary excretion of sodium because of a direct inhibitory effect on sodium transport in the inner medullary collecting duct.

MANAGEMENT

- Treatment of the underlying neurologic problem
- Volume replacement with isotonic saline or oral salt suppressing release of vasopressin The recommended correction rate is 0.7 to 1.0 mmol/L per hour, with a maximum of 8 to 10 mmol/L per 24 hours.
- Fludrocortisone an aldosterone receptor agonist, produce volume expansion and sodium retention, but the potassium concentration and blood pressure should be monitored. Dose is 50 to 100 microgram daily.

The duration of CSW is usually 3 to 5 weeks. The differentiation from SIADH is important though difficult.

Fluid restriction is the cornerstone therapy for SIADH, whereas as fluid correction is treatment of choice in CSW.

Nephrogenic Syndrome of Inappropriate Antidiuresis

Abnormality is identified as mutation of v_2 receptor. The diagnostic criteria is same as for SIADH, but *ADH levels are below detectable limits.*

TURP SYNDROME

This is defined as plasma Na less than 125 mmol/L., with two or more associated clinical signs or symptoms. The symptoms can be masked under general anesthesia. Syndrome similar to this has also been reported in females undergoing transcervical endometrial ablation and in patients undergoing neuroendoscopic ventriculostomy.

Neurological symptoms develop when Na falls below 123 mmol/L and cardiac symptoms below 100 mmol/L. Incidence of TURP syndrome is decreasing with the use of glycine as an irrigant.

Pathophysiology

This is due to the absorption of irrigant solutions directly through the prostatic venous plexuses or more slowly from the retroperitoneal and perivesical space.

Risk Factors are
  a. Open prostatic venous sinuses
  b. High irrigation pressure > 30 mm Hg
  c. Hypotonic irrigants
  d. Large volume of irrigant
  e. Resection time > one hour

  Sequelae TURP Syndrome

Large volumes of irrigants can get absorbed into the vascular compartment and dilute the sodium of ECF. The blood loss during surgery and treatment with diuretics can precipitate hyponatremia. There can be ECF volume expansion which can result in fluid over load, cardiac failure and acute pulmonary edema. Patient can present with symptoms due to hyponatremia- Cerebral edema. If glycine is used this may result in encephalopathy from ammonia accumulation (Fig. 4.12).

TURP syndrome can also result in AKI and is caused by hypotension and hypoperfusion to the kidneys. This is due to capillary leak and blood loss during surgery. This results in low GFR. Spinal anesthesia may rarely cause hypotension. Hyponatremia in TURP syndrome can result in hemolysis and contribute to AKI (Fig. 4.13).

Management of TURP Syndrome

- Mainstay is prevention of development of TURP
- Keep irrigation pressure less than 15 cm H_2O
- Resection time should be kept less than 1 hour

Na should be monitored frequently and correction of hyponatremia is as per guidelines.

Primary Polydipsia

Primary polydipsia is associated with excessive thirst resulting in increased water intake. This excessive water intake can dilute

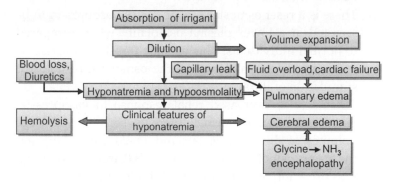

Fig. 4.12: Sequelae TURP syndrome

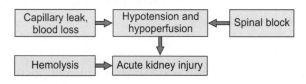

Fig. 4.13: Pathogenesis of acute kidney injury (AKI)

the ECF volume and result in hyponatremia. This is usually seen in patients with psychiatric disorders and hyponatremia in such situations is intermittent. Hence, this is also described as intermittent hyponatremia polydipsia syndrome.

Antipsychotic drugs cause dry mouth leading to increase in water intake. This can cause hyponatremia.

Pathophysiology

There is increased water intake. Water retention is inappropriate to plasma osmolality.

Causes for Increased Water Intake

Causes for water retention—Different types of abnormalities in ADH regulation are described.

1. Increase in thirst perception occurs at lower plasma osmolality when compared to normal individuals.
2. The antipsychotic medications cause dry mouth which leads to increase in water intake.
3. There is a reset osmostat which causes vasopressin to be secreted at a lower plasma osmolality when compared to normal individuals. This osmotic threshold for release of vasopressin is higher than the osmotic threshold for stimulation of thirst.
4. There is also decreased renal response to vasopressin. Since kidneys are normal, there is secretion of large volumes of dilute urine [around 15–20 liters/day] and the urine osmolality is usually < 100 milliosmoles/kg. This excretion of large volume of dilute urine protects the patient from fluid overload states. Here the ADH levels are low and should be differentiated from SIADH where ADH levels are high.

Treatment

Main stay is restriction of water intake. This will increase the plasma sodium concentration.

EXERCISE-ASSOCIATED HYPONATREMIA (EAH)

This is described in long distance marathon runners.

Risk factors for hyponatremia in EAH are:

* Low body mass index
* Race time > 4 hours
* Consumption of fluid every mile because they are instructed to drink as much as possible during the race
* Increased frequency of micturition during the race
* Use of NSAIDS
* ? Females

Pathophysiology of EAH

Development of hyponatremia is due to dilution of sodium in larger volume of water.

Increased volume of water results from (Fig. 4.14):

1. Increased water intake because long distance runners are instructed to take fluids frequently.
2. Exercise causes increase in cellular metabolism resulting in increased production of water.
3. Stress, exercise, inadequate fluid intake, and cytokine release can result in ADH release causing water retention.
4. Inadequate intake of fluids can result in hypovolemia, reduction in renal blood flow resulting in reduction of GFR which in turn results in decreased delivery of solutes to distal tubules.
5. There is also inability to mobilize sodium from the stores causing hyponatremia.

Hyponatremia in such situations can persist beyond the completion of exercise. This is due to absorption of large amount of retained hypotonic fluids in the GI tract.

MANAGEMENT

* Suspect EAH in any athlete who present with symptoms suggestive of hyponatremia

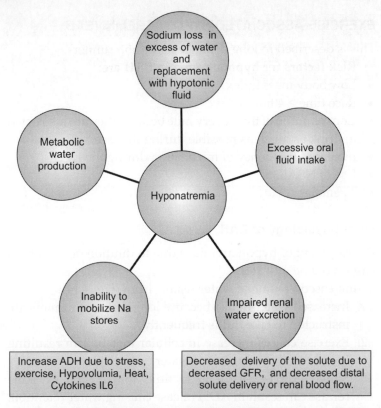

Fig. 4.14: Pathophysiology of EAH

Asymptomatic Mild Hyponatremia [130–135 millimoles/L]

Treatment is fluid restriction. Patient should be observed with frequent monitoring of serum sodium and potassium till the development of spontaneous diuresis.

Indication for Normal Saline

Normal Saline is indicated in athletes who have clinical signs of hypovolemia and serum sodium should be frequently monitored. Injudicious administration of normal saline can result in fluid overload and pulmonary edema. Symptomatic EAH with serum sodium less than 120 millimloes/L should be managed with hypertonic saline.

Caution: Sudden correction of hypovolemia can suppress ADH resulting in correction of sodium to a value greater than expected by infusion of saline alone. When hyponatremia develops within 48 hours of exercise, it is considered as acute. Treatment consist of 3% of saline given at a rate of 1–2 mL/kg/h and serum sodium potassium, urinary sodium and urinary potassium should be regulary monitored. If urine volume does not increase, the rate of infusion can be increased to 2–4 mL/kg/h. When free water excretion increases, the rate of infusion should be decreased or infusion should be stopped depending on sodium value. Athletes who develop confusion, vomiting, respiratory insufficiency are considered to have severe hyponatremia.

Treatment - 100 mL of 3% saline should be infused rapidly over 10 minutes. This will raise the serum sodium by 2–3 millimoles/L.

Loop diuretics are indicated in
1. Significant volume overload and
2. Significant antidiuresis with elevated urinary osmolality, sodium, and/or potassium level.

Correction of Hypokalemia

Hypokalemia usually develops in athletes after completion of the athletic event. Hypokalemia associated with hyponatremia should be corrected. Correction of hypokalemia corrects sodium deficit by exit of sodium from the cells.

There is no role for vasopressin antagonist in EAH.

Osmotic demyelination syndrome is not reported with rapid correction of sodium in EAH.

POTOMANIA (EXCESSIVE BEER INGESTION)

Does not usually cause significant hyponatremia because the normal kidney has a marked ability to excrete dilute urine. When hyponatremia is detected in these conditions, exclude additional/superadded problem preventing the urine from being maximally dilute due to either ADH release, drugs, volume contraction due to vomiting, diuretics, an associated physical illness/stress or an impaired ability to excrete free water due to an associated glucocorticoid/thyroid hormone deficiency.

IN NEONATES AND CHILDREN

In children 70% of body weight is water. As in adults, Hypotonic hyponatremia is classified based on ECF volume. ECF volume deficit is considered to be mild when there is less than 3% decrease in body weight, moderate with 3–6% decrease, severe when there is more than 6% decrease in body weight. More than 9% decrease is considered an emergency.

If the clinical problem has developed within 48 hours, this is considered acute. Fluid losses are derived from the ECF and ICF in the ratio 80:20%. If the duration is more than 48 hours fluid losses are derived from the ECF and ICF in the ratio 60:40%.

In isotonic fluid losses sodium can be calculated by multiplying **140 × ECF portion of the loss**.

Potassium deficit can be calculated by multiplying **140 mmol/L × ICF losses**.

Case History 9

An 18-month-old child developed diarrhea. Present weight is 10 kg and has lost 5% of body weight. How is fluid requirement calculated?

Total fluid requirement is
Fluid required for deficit correction + maintenance requirement.
If there is any ongoing loss that should also be corrected.

Calculation of Fluid Deficit

Assessed fluid loss is 500 ml.

Since fluid loss is acute, the ECF: ICF ratio is 80:20

$$\text{ECF loss} = 80\% = \frac{80}{100} \times 500 \text{ mL} = 400 \text{ mL}$$

$$ICF \ deficit = 20\% = \frac{20}{100} \times 500 \ mL = 100 \ mL$$

Na deficit = **140 mmol/L** × ECF portion of the loss
= 140 × 400 = **56 mmol**

K deficit = **140 mmol/L** × ICF losses.

$$=140 \times \frac{100}{1000} = \textbf{14 mmol.}$$

Volume of fluid required for deficit correction is 500 mL and should contain 56 mmoles of sodium and 14 mmoles of potassium.

Calculation of Maintenance Requirement

Daily fluid requirement = 100 mL/kg till 10 kg = 1000 mL.

Na = 3 mmol for every 100 mL = 30 mmol and
K = 2 mmol for every 100 mL = 20 mmol

Total requirement = Fluid Deficit + maintenance requirement
= 1000 + 500 mL = 1500 mL

Na requirement = 56 + 30 = 86 mmol/L
K requirement = 14 + 20 = 34 mmol.

Ideal fluid will be ½ normal saline with 17 mL of KCl added and should be run in 24 hours. Ongoing losses also have to be replaced. Guidelines for correction are the same as in adults.

COMPLICATIONS OF RAPID CORRECTION

Osmotic Demyelination Syndrome (ODS)

This is a life threatening of complication of rapid correction of hyponatremia. Previously called as central pontine myelinolysis was first described by Victor and Adams in 1959. Aggressive correction exceeding the permitted rate of correction and total rise of Na can produce ODS. This is associated with high morbidity and mortality than uncorrected hyponatremia itself.

Risk Factors are:
- Alcoholism
- Malnutrition,
- Patients with burns;

- Severe potassium depletion—It is possible that the failure to replete brain potassium may not allow these patients to osmoregulate well in the brain.
- Elderly women on thiazide diuretics (present acutely, or can also present 3 to 5 days later)
- Adrenal insufficiency
- Cerebral edema
- HIV

Sites involved are pons, internal capsule, cerebellum, cerebrum

Clinical features—depend on the site affected. May present with quadriparesis, quadriplegia, dysarthria, tremor, seizures, locked in syndrome.

MANAGEMENT

The damage is irreversible. Main stay is to prevent over-correction of hyponatremia. When Na is replaced too rapidly (e.g., > 14 mmol/L/8 h) and neurologic symptoms develop, it is critical to prevent further increases in serum Na by stopping hypertonic fluids. Hypotonic fluids like 5% dextrose should be infused to bring back sodium to safe levels.

KEY POINTS

- True hyponatremia is always associated with hypo-osmolality.
- Hyponatremia can be associated with low, normal or high ECF volume.
- GFR should be calculated.
- Urine sodium less than 10 mmol/L indicate extrarenal losses and more than 20 mmol/L renal losses.
- Urine potassium estimation, will give a clue to the diagnosis.
- Hypovolemic hypontaremia should be corrected with saline replacement after assessing ECF volume deficit.
- Euvolemic hyponatremia SIADH, mainstay is fluid restriction.
- If ECF volume is expanded, use of frusemide and replacement of urinary loss of Na in lesser volume of

water may help. Dialysis is indicated in diuretic resistant pulmonary edema.

- Hyponatremia should be corrected aggressively only if this has developed within 48 hours and is causing neurological symptoms or plasma Na less than 110 mmol/L.
- Rate of rise of Na should be 8–12 mmol/L in 24 hours.
- ODS is an ominous complication and should be prevented.

Summary of clinical approach to hyponatremia is shown in Figure 4.15.

Therapeutic Approach to hypotonic hyponatremia s shown in Figure 4.16

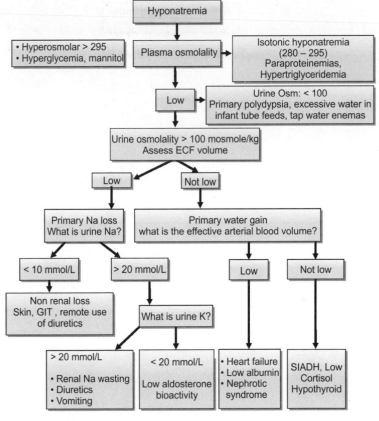

Fig. 4.15: Summary of clinical approach to hypernatremia

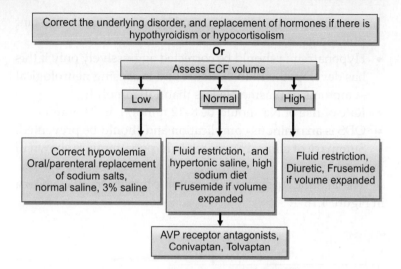

Fig. 4.16: Therapeutic approach to hypotonic hyponatremia

CHAPTER

5

Hypernatremia

A Vimala

OVERVIEW

Hypernatremia is defined as plasma Na > 145 mmol/L and is diagnosed as severe when Na is more than 150 mmol/L in children and 160 mmol/L in adults. Hypernatremia is rare and is seen in extremes of age. Plasma sodium (Na) above 145 mmol/L is always associated with hyperosmolar state and decrease in cell volume - **cellular dehydration**. This is responsible for the symptoms and signs of hypernatremia. Rapid correction of hypernatremia can produce cerebral edema. Formulae are available for calculating the volume of hypotonic fluid/free water required for correction.

WHAT IS HYPERNATREMIA?

As discussed in the earlier chapter, abnormalities in sodium homeostasis are always due to altered water handling. Plasma Sodium concentration is derived by dividing total body Na in mmol/L by total body water in liters.

$$\frac{Na\ (mmol/L)}{TBW}$$

The pathogenesis of hypernatremia is hypotonic fluid loss, pure water loss or gain of sodium. The most common cause is hypotonic fluid loss which is corrected with electrolyte rich solution and inadequate pure water replacement.

Hypotonic Fluid Loss

Scenario 1: If 20 mmol of Na and 300 mL of water is lost from one liter of solution containing 140 millimoles of sodium/L New Na concentration will be $120/700 \times 1000 = 171$ mmol/L.

Pure Water Loss

Scenario 2: When 300 mL of water is lost from one liter of solution containing 140 millimoles of sodium/L, the new sodium concentration will be $140/700 \times 1000 = 200$ mmol/L.

Increased Sodium Load

Scenario 3: If 50 mL of 0.9% sodium bicarbonate solution is infused there is gain of 45 mmol of sodium, the new Na will be 185 mmol/1050 mL = 176 mmol/L.

Thus, it can be seen that hypernatremia can be due to:

- *Hypotonic fluid losses i.e. water more than sodium can be lost through renal or extrarenal route.*
- *Net loss of water and sodium from the body with inadequate water replacement (most common cause).*
- *Increased Sodium Load – infusion of hypertonic infusions containing sodium.*

Pure Water Deficit

The most common cause of pure water deficit is excessive evaporative loss of water through skin and respiratory tract. When there is a hypotonic fluid loss this should be corrected with fluid rich in water – similar in composition to the fluid that is lost. Water loss can be due to loss of hypotonic fluids which is (common in children) due to reduced action of anti-diuretic hormone (ADH). ADH secretion can be reduced due to diseases of hypothalamus, pituitary or diminished response of collecting duct to ADH. Drugs mainly osmotic diuretics and diseases of the renal interstitium can impair free water clearance and result in hypernatremia.

Net Loss of Water and Sodium from the Body with Inadequate Water Replacement

Suppose there is a hypotonic loss of fluid from ECF. The composition of the fluid lost is 300 mL of water containing 30 millimoles of sodium. If electrolyte solutions like normal saline are used, 300 mL normal saline contain 46 millimoles of sodium chloride. This will distribute more sodium in less water and can give rise to hypernatremia. This hypotonic fluid loss should be replaced with a solution which contain 100 millimoles/L of sodium chloride.

Increased Sodium Load

Hypertonic infusions containing sodium (Sodium bicarbonate infusions, hypertonic saline), give additional sodium to plasma resulting in gain of sodium.

Why Recognize Hypernatremia?

- Acute severe hypernatremia can cause substantial morbidity and mortality due to neurological complications.
- This is a predictor of bad prognosis in critically ill patients
- Rapid correction of chronic hypernatremia can cause severe neurologic deficits and death.

Mild hypernatremia does not produce symptoms.

Pathophysiology

As plasma sodium increases, plasma osmolality increases. This creates an osmotic pressure difference between ICF and ECF. Normally Na concentration is very low in the cells. Na diffuses in to the cell along the concentration and electrical gradient. Na that enters the cell is pumped out of the cell through basolateral membrane $Na^+/K^+/ATPase$. In order to attain osmotic equilibrium, water flows from ICF to ECF and Intracellular dehydration occurs.

Scenario 4: In a 50-year-old male plasma sodium is 160 mmol/L. His weight is 60 kg. Find out the ICF fluid deficit? (Fig. 5.1)

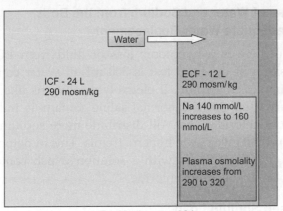

Total body water 36 L

Fig. 5.1: Changes in ECF osmolality in scenario 4

Normal plasma Na = 140 mmol/L
Normal ICF osmolality = ECF osmolality = 290 mosm/kg
Total body water = 60% of body weight = 36L
ICF water = 40% = 24L, ECF water = 20% = 12L
With increase in plasma Na to 160 mmol/L,
ECF osmolality = ICF osmolality = 160 × 2 = 320 mosm/kg
Since there is no change in ICF solutes, the increase in osmolality is
due to decrease in water
ICF osmolality = (Normal ICF osmolality × ICF volume
= 290 × 24 = 6960
Current ICF osmolality = 320 mosm/kg
Current ICF water = 6960/320 = 21.75 L.
ICF deficit = 24 – 21.75 = 2.25L)
Cells have lost 2.25 Liters of water.

This new osmotic equilibrium results in cellular dehydration. *Hyperosmolality can result in cellular dehydration and cell shrinkage.* The shrinkage of brain can lead to stretching of blood vessels resulting in rupture and hemorrhages.

In chronic hypernatremia, to prevent cellular dehydration electrolytes will be transported from ECF to ICF. In addition there is synthesis of new intracellular osmolytes in 24–48 hours. This will create a new osmotic equilibrium but at a higher osmolality. If hypernatremia is rapidly corrected with hypotonic fluid, the ECF osmolality will decrease. Since ICF has higher osmolality, water will move in to the cells and cause cerebral oedema.

CLINICAL FEATURES

Hypernatremia is rare and reported in only 0.5 to 5% of hospitalized patients. Morbidity and mortality is more in geriatric age group when compared to adults. The mortality rate for severe acute hypernatremia in the ICU setting is as high as 75% in contrast to chronic hypernatremia where it is only 10%. Incidence of hypernatremia is increased in people with certain risk factors.

Risk Factors for Development of Hypernatremia in the Community

1. Extremes of age
2. Underlying neurological disorders
3. Primary hypodipsia
4. Diabetes mellitus
5. Diabetes insipidus and other polyuric states

Risk Factors Identified in Hospitalized Patients

1. Tube-feeding with concentrated solutions and less of free water — Hypertonic solutions
2. Use of osmotic diuretics usually given for cerebral edema,
3. Lactulose — Produces osmotic diarrhea when more free water is lost.
4. Mechanical ventilation.

Signs and Symptoms of Hypernatremia

Hypernatremia is acute if there is a normal documented Na+ value within 48 hours of detecting hypernatremia. If the rise in sodium occurs in more than 48 hours, it is chronic. Symptoms depend on absolute level of sodium. Patients become symptomatic when sodium exceeds 160 millimoles/L.

Gradual slow rise in sodium does not produce any symptoms. The symptoms of hypernatremia can be nonspecific or due to neurological complications. Non-specific symptoms are fever and nausea. If the thirst center is intact, hyperosmolality will stimulate the thirst center leading to increased water intake. This is a physiological mechanism to correct hypernatremia. Patients can also present with polyuria.

Hypernatremic Encephalopathy

The dangerous squeale to hypernatremia is hypernatremic encephalopathy. They can present with symptoms directly attributable to hypernatremia. This can range

- From thirst (if thirst centre is intact), confusion, irritability, alteration of sensorium, muscle spasm and hyperreflexia.
- Seizures can be a clinical presentation, especially in children
- Severe hypernatremia can result in coma and death.

Pathophysiology

Normal compensatory mechanism to restore ECF volume are
1. Decrease in GFR
2. Increase in reabsorption of sodium and water from proximal convoluted tubule (PCT), and distal tubule
3. Decrease in free water clearance by action of ADH in the collecting duct
4. Stimulation of thirst center and increase in water intake.

Restoration of ECF volume will prevent the development of hypernatremia. Hypernatremia will develop when the physiological mechanisms fail.
1. Decrease in water intake
2. Failure of renal compensatory mechanisms.

Decrease in Water Intake

If thirst center is destroyed due to disease, or patient has restricted access to free water, hypernatremia will develop. This can also occur when patients are fed through Ryle's tube with concentrated solutions. When there is net loss of water (with more of water than sodium) and the losses are replaced with inadequate free water. Patients can develop hypernatremia.

Hypernatremia due to inadequate water intake is rarely seen in alert patients with a normal thirst mechanism and access to water.

Failure of Renal Compensatory Mechanisms

This is due to defective handling of sodium and increase in free water excretion as in interstitial diseases of the kidney, due to defective action of ADH on the collecting duct.

Inadequate water intake is a universal prerequisite for the evolution of hypernatremia

CLASSIFICATION AND APPROACH

Classified based on ECF volume into hypovolemic, euvolemic and hypervolemic hypernatremia (Fig. 5.2).

The following steps will help to evaluate hypernatremia

Step 1: Assessment of ECF volume

Step 2: Measurement of urine osmolality and urine sodium

Step 3: Compare urine osmolality to plasma osmolality

Step 4: Measure urine sodium, potassium, chloride and compare to urine osmolality.

Step 5: If urine $(Na^+ + K^+) < Cl^-$, measure urine PH

First step is clinical assessment of ECF volume

Step 1: Hypovolemia assessment ECF volume

Signs of ECF volume depletion are described in Figure 5.3

Loss of 1 g of weight = 1 mL of fluid

Signs of ECF Volume Expansion

Increase in JVP, edema and ascites.

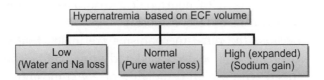

Fig. 5.2: Classification of hypernatremia based on ECF volume

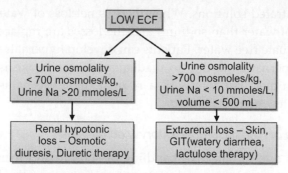

Fig. 5.3: Causes of hypernatremia with low ECF volume

Hypovolemic Hypernatremia

Can result *from loss of water more than electrolytes (hypotonic fluid losses) or pure water deficit.*

Approach to Hypovolemic Hypernatremia

A good history will give a clue to the cause of hypovolemia. Signs of ECF volume depletion and grading into mild, moderate and severe is shown in Table 5.1. The following steps are used in further evaluation.

Measure urine osmolality and urine sodium.

1. **High urine osmolality of > 700 mosmoles/kg and low urine Na < 10 mmol/L-**
   Usual causes are (Fig. 5.3)
   a. Low ECF volume due to extrarenal cause.
      Loss of fluid through skin and respiratory tract losses in hot environment during exercise, febrile patients, patients on mechanical ventilation.
   b. *Inadequate water intake* usually seen in extremes of age, in patients with neurological disorders, in primary hypodipsia, or reset osmostat.
      Because the renal mechanisms are intact, free water clearance will be decreased and urine will be concentrated with a high osmolality of > 700 mosmoles/kg and low urine Na < 10 mmol/L.

Table 5.1: Signs of ECF volume depletion

Findings	Mild	Moderate	Severe
Pulse	Normal	Rapid	Rapid and weak
BP	Normal	Postural hypotension	Persistent hypotension
Weight loss	< 5%	10%	> 15%
Infants	< 3%	5–6%	9–10%
Others			
Mucosa	Tacky	Dry	Parched
Skin turgor	Mild decrease	Decreased	Tenting
Eyes	Normal tearing	Decreased tearing sunken	No tears, sunken
Capillary refill	Normal	Delayed > 3 sec	Delayed > 5 sec
Urine output	Low	< 500 mL (0.5 mL/kg/h)	Anuric

2. **Low urine osmolality of < 700 mosm/kg and high urine Na > 20 mmol/L (Fig. 5.3).**

   This is seen when there is increase excretion of osmoles in urine and when volume of urine is increased

   Causes are

   a. *Osmotic diuresis – Glycosuria,* high urea excretion, use of osmotic diuretics like Mannitol.

   b. Administration of loop diuretics, thiazides, etc. leading to increase in volume.

3. **Very low urine osmolality of < 150 mosm/kg and variable sodium excretion**

   a. This is due to defective/reduced or absent secretion of anti-diuretic hormone (ADH).

   b. Inability of renal tubules to respond to ADH.

Case History 1

A-75-year-old gentleman was admitted in a confused state. There was no significant past illness, was started on statins recently. On clinical examination, he has no loss of weight. He was tachycardic, BP 110/70 mm Hg (baseline BP 130/90 mm Hg), diminished skin turgor and muscles were tender.

Laboratory parameters are as follows

Parameter	Value
RBS	90 mg%
Creatinine	1.1 mg%
Urea	65 mg%
Sodium	180 mmol/L
Potassium	3.5 mmol/L

This patient has disproportionate elevation of urea, and severe hypernatremia.

Step 1: *Assessment of ECF volume*
Patient has clinical evidence of ECF volume contraction.

Step 2: Measure urine volume, urine osmolality, urine sodium

Parameter	Value
Urine volume	300 mL in 24 hours
Urine Na	10 mmol/L
Urine osmolality	1200 mosmoles/kg

Kidneys are responding appropriately by reabsorption of water as shown by low urine volume, high urine osmolality and low urine sodium.

Alteration of sensorium suggests that there is loss of water from brain cells. ECF volume contraction with *no documented loss of weight* indicates that contraction is not because of external loss of water.

Other investigations were

Parameter	Value
Plasma Ca	7.5 mg/dL
plasma PO_4	8 mg/dL
Serum albumin	4 g/L
CPK	3500 units

These findings suggested rhabdomyolysis. ECF volume contraction was due to shift of water into muscles.
Hypernatremia in this patient is due to ECF volume contraction. Here there is shift of water from ECF to muscles. Hence, there was no change in weight.

Hypernatremia and Normal ECF

This is usually due to pure water deficit. Pure water deficit can be due to increased free water clearance as in diabetes insipidus or increased insensible loss. Patients with primary or secondary hypodipsia can also develop hypernatremia. The appropriate renal response in high plasma osmolality is high urine osmolality. This indicates that ADH is acting normally and renal mechanisms are in tact. Hence renal and extra renal causes can be differentiated by measuring urine osmolality.

Step 1: To measure urine volume and urine osmolality
High urine osmolality of > 700 mosmoles/kg
Causes are diminished water intake due to primary or secondary hypodipsia and or increased insensible loss.

- *Low urine osmolality of < 700 mosmoles/kg*
  Free water clearance is under the influence of ADH. Defective urinary concentration points to diabetes insipidus (DI). To differentiate central DI from nephrogenic DI, ADH infusion is given. Increase in urine osmolality after ADH infusion is suggestive of central DI (Fig. 5.4).

Hypernatremia and ECF Volume Expansion

Additional infusion of hypertonic sodium containing infusions of Nacl, Na HCO_3, or increased intake of oral salt can result in hypernatremia. This is a very rare cause (Fig. 5.5).

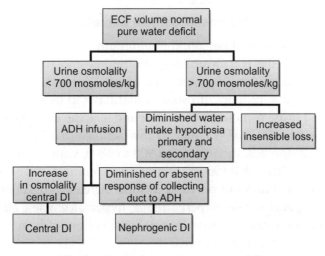

Fig. 5.4: Approach based on urine osmolality

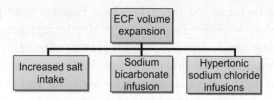

Fig. 5.5: Causes of hypernatremia due to ECF volume expansion

Polyuria

One of the most important symptoms of hypernatremia is polyuria. Polyuria can be defined as urine volume more than 1.5 to 2 mL/kg/h in children and more than 2.5 L/day in adults. Normal urine volume is determined by the total osmoles that have to be excreted and the free water clearance.

Urine volume = volume required for osmole excretion + free water clearance.

So polyuria can occur when there is an increase in osmole excretion or increase in free water clearance. Urine osmolality will increase with increase in osmole excretion or with decrease in free water excretion.

Polyuria due to Increased Osmole Excretion

In a resting normal person, the minimum daily osmotic load to be excreted is 600 mosmloles. Minimum osmolality that can be attained is 50 milliosmoles and urine volume can increase to 600 ÷ 50 = 12 liters. If osmoles that have to be excreted is 900 and urine osmolality is also around 900, the urine volume required is 900/900 = 1 liter. If the osmoles that have to be excreted doubles, increase from 900 to 1800, volume of urine required will be 1800/900 = 2 liters. Causes for increased osmole excretion resulting in polyuria include increased excretion of urea, hyperglycemia, hypernatremia, hypercalcemiaetc etc.

Let us see how increase in metabolism of muscle can result in increased excretion of urea.

Metabolism of 1 kg of muscle can increase osmotic load from 900 to 1800 osmoles. This is based on the following calculation 100 gm of muscle tissue contains 80% water and 20% protein. Hence 1000 g (1 kg) will contain 200 g of protein.
100 g of protein contains 16 gm of nitrogen.
200 g of protein contains 32 g nitrogen. 1000 g of muscle which has 200 g of protein will produce 32 g of nitrogen.

To Find out the Urea Required to Excrete 32 G of Nitrogen

60 gm (1 mole) of urea contains 28 g nitrogen (molecular formula of urea is NH_2- CO -NH_2) i.e. to produce 32 g nitrogen, urea required is $32/28 \times 60 = 68.5$ gms of urea = 1.143 moles of urea. Hence, metabolism of 1 kg muscle will lead to additional excretion of urea.

Polyuria due to Decreased Urine Osmolality

The second cause of polyuria can be defective concentration capacity of medullary interstitium due to drugs or diseases. Here ADH action is normal. Hence urine osmolality is close to that of plasma osmolality of 300.

Approach to Polyuria

Diagnostic approach to polyuria starts with measurement of urine and plasma osmolality. Urine osmolality less than 150 milliosmoles/kg indicate diabetes Insipidus (DI) or excessive water ingestion as in psychogenic polydipsia.

Urine osmolality equal to or more than plasma osmolality indicate medullary wash out of solutes, osmotic diuresis or increased excretion of electrolytes in urine (Fig. 5.6).

Approach to Polyuria Based on Osmolality

This is based on measurement of sodium (Na), potassium (K) , chloride (Cl-) and osmolality of urine (Fig. 5.7).

As mentioned earlier polyuria can occur with increased osmole excretion. This is suggested by high urine osmolality

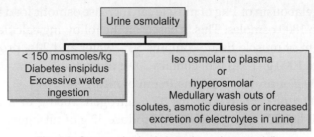

Fig. 5.6: Causes of polyuria based on urine osmolality

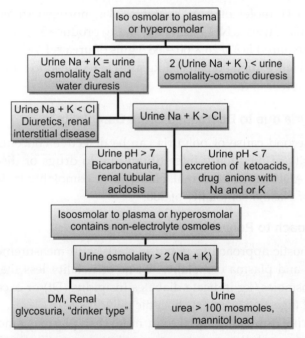

Fig. 5.7: Approach to hypernatremia in isoosmolar or hyperosmolar urine based on urine Na, K estimation

which can be equal to or more than plasma osmolality. The normal urine osmolality is due to excretion of sodium and potassium. In hyperosmolar urine,

1. **Step 1: If urine osmolality = 2 × (urine Na + urine K),** This suggest there is increased excretion of sodium and potassium in urine. This can be due to diuretic therapy,

interstitial nephritis (defective secretion of NH_4), excretion of anions like keto acids or drug anions

Step 2: Calculate urine anion gap. Urine anion gap = Urine (Na + K) – Cl^-, if urine (Na^+ + K^+) is < Cl^-, probable causes are diuretic therapy, or interstitial nephritis

If Urine (Na + K) is more than Cl^- to find out the cause, measure urine pH. Urine pH more than 7 indicates defective secretion of NH_4, and presence of bicarbonate (HCO_3) in urine.

2. **Urine osmolality is more than 2 × (urine Na + urine K)** Presence of non-electrolyte solutes like glucose, urea or mannitol in urine is suggested.

   Urine pH less than 7 indicates excretion of anions like keto acids or drug anions in urine

Approach to Polyuria Based on Osmolality

Case History 2

A 65-year-old man developed hemiplegia, and was aphasic. He was fed through Ryle's tube and was discharged. 7 days later he was readmitted in a stuporous state. There was no focal neurological deficit. He was hypovolemic. Urine volume was around 4 liters.

Laboratory parameters are as follows

Parameter	Value
RBS	100 mg%
Creatinine	1.1 mg%
Urea	40 mg%
Sodium	150 mmol/L
Potassium	4 mmol/L
Plasma osmolality	312 mosm/kg

This patient has polyuria, severe hypernatremia, disproportionate elevation of urea. Hypernatremia is evaluated as follows:

Step 1: Assessment of ECF volume

Patient has evidence of low ECF volume.

Step 2: Measurement of urine osmolality and urine sodium

Parameter	Value
Urine volume	4 L in 24 hours
Urine Na	120 mmol/L
Urine K	40 mm0/L
Urine osmolality	500 mosm/K

Urine osmolality is 500 milliosmoles and sodium and K excretion is 120 millimoles/L and 40 mmoles/L respectively.

Step 3: Compare urine osmolality to plasma osmolality

Patient has high urine osmolality compared to plasma. This indicates that polyuria is due to increased excretion of osmotically active particles in urine. Na and K are the usual solutes contributing to urine osmolality.

Step 4: Calculate urine osmolality using the formula 2 × (urine sodium + potassium), and compare with measured urine osmolality

Calculated urine osmolality = 2 × (120 + 40) = 320.

Measured osmolality = 500 milliosmoles/kg

Measured osmolality is greater than calculated osmolality and this suggests presence of osmotic solutes other than sodium and potassium in urine

Step 5: *Test for other osmotic solutes.* There is no history of administration of osmotic agents or diabetes mellitus.

Blood sugar was normal. Hence, the other important osmotic solute — urea was measured. Urine urea = > 400mg/day suggesting increased excretion of urea. High urine urea in this patient was derived from the high protein feeds. *Management* — Patient was given 2/3rd of the total requirement as free water. Hypernatremia was corrected by infusion of 5% dextrose.

Diabetes Insipidus (DI)

Diabetes insipidus *is* a syndrome characterized by the production of abnormally large volumes of dilute urine. The 24h urine volume should be more than 50 mL/kg body weight and the osmolality should be less than 300 mosmol/kg.

Vasopressin (Arginine Vasopressin - AVP)

Normal site of production of vasopressin (Arginine vasopressin-AVP) also known as Anti-diuretic hormone (ADH) is neuro-hypophysis, which is formed by axons that originate in large cell bodies in the supraoptic and paraventricular nuclei of the hypothalamus. ADH released into blood is transported to the receptor site on the basolateral surface of the collecting duct membrane. This antidiuretic effect is achieved by increasing the hydroosmotic permeability of cells that line the distal tubule and medullary collecting ducts of the kidney by increasing the exocytic insertion of *Aquaporin*. The actions of ADH are mediated through at least 2 receptors:

V 1 mediates vasoconstriction, enhancement of corticotrophin release, and renal prostaglandin synthesis;

V2 mediates the antidiuretic response. Water is reabsorbed by osmotic equilibration with the hypertonic interstitium and returned to the systemic circulation.

Role of Arginine Vasopressin (AVP) in the Regulation of Urine Volume

Normal GFR in a normal adult is 180 Liters. 144 L (60%) of GFR is reabsorbed in the proximal tubule by isoosmotic reabsorption, another 8 L (4–5%) is reabsorbed without solute in the descending limb of Henle's loop. In the ascending limb, there is selective reabsorption of sodium and chloride. Water is reabsorbed in the distal tubule and collecting duct, In the presence of AVP, medullary interstitium is hypertonic. Solute-free water is reabsorbed osmotically through the principal cells of the collecting ducts, and is mediated by ADH. This results in the excretion of small volume of concentrated urine. This antidiuretic effect is mediated via a G protein-coupled V_2 receptor that increases intracellular cyclic AMP. This induces translocation of aquaporin 2 (AQP 2) water channels into the apical membrane and increases the efflux of water into the cells.

AQP 3 and AQP 4 water channels on the basolateral surface shifts water into systemic circulation.

The main determinants of water movement are the number of AQP 2 water channels in the apical membrane and the strength of the osmotic gradient between tubular fluid and the renal medulla

Stimuli for release are increase in plasma osmolality due to increase in Na only and hypovolemia. In the absence of AVP, these cells are impermeable to water and results in the excretion of very large volumes as much as 0.2 mL/kg per minute of maximally dilute urine 1.000 and 50 mosmol/kg, (specific gravity and osmolality respectively), a condition known as a *water diuresis.*

Classification of Diabetes Insipidus (DI)

Central DI — Failure of release of ADH in response to high plasma osmolality

Nephrogenic DI — Inadequate or absent response of the cortical and medullary collecting tubules to ADH.

Causes are shown in the Table 5.2.

Table 5.2: Cause of diabetes insipidus

Central DI	Nephrogenic DI
• *Idiopathic DI* — auto immune following surgery-cranio-pharyngioma or pineal tumors • *Trauma,* base of skull fractures • *Infections* — Meningitis, encephalitis • *Neoplasms* of brain, lung cancer, lymphoma, leukemia) • *Hypoxic encephalopathy* • *Infiltrative disorders* (histiocytosis X, sarcoidosis • *Vascular lesions* — Arterio venous malformations, aneurysma • *Drugs* — phenytoin • *Familial*	Acquired *Drugs* — Lithium, demeclocycline, methoxyflurane amphotericin B aminoglycosides cisplatin *Metabolic* — Hypokalemia, hypercalcemia, hypercalciuria obstruction (ureter or urethra) *Vascular* — Sickle cell disease and trait Ischemia (acute tubular necrosis) granulomas primary polydipsia *Genetic* X-linked recessive (AVP receptor-2 gene) autosomal recessive (aquaporin-2 gene) autosomal dominant (aquaporin-2 gene *Miscellaneous* — pregnancy, neoplasms, idiopathic, iatrogenic

Symptoms

Increase in urinary frequency, enuresis, and/or nocturia, which may disturb sleep and cause mild daytime fatigue or somnolence. If the thirst center is intact, this will be stimulated. There is increase in fluid intake (polydipsia) and will prevent dehydration.

Criteria to diagnose Diabetes insipidus

- ECF volume is normal/can be low
- Plasma sodium is high normal > 160 mmol/L (If thirst mechanism is intact, increase in water intake will keep Na in upper limit of normal).
- Plasma osmolality > 320 mOsm/kg
- Signs of dehydration especially in infants
- A urine specific gravity of 1.005 or less and a urine osmolality less than 200 mosm/kg.

Treatment

- Encourage to drink enough free water to replace their urine losses.
- Intravenous dextrose or IV fluid that is hypoosmolar to the patient's serum.

Precautions; avoid hyperglycemia, volume overload, and overly rapid correction of hypernatremia.

Rule of thumb is to reduce serum sodium by 0.5 mmol/L/h.

Case History 3

A 25-year-old lady was admitted with history polyuria. Clinically, she was euvolemic. Systemic examination was unremarkable.

Laboratory parameters are as follows:

Parameter	value
RBS	95 mg%
Creatinine	1.1 mg%
Urea	25 mg%
Sodium	145 mmol/L
Plasma osmolality	300 mosm/kg

She had polyuria, normal GFR with plasma sodium and osmolality in the upper limit of normal.

Step 1: Assessment of ECF volume—Patient was euvolemic.

Step 2: Measure urine osmolality and urine sodium, urine specific gravity.

Parameter	Value
Urine volume	6 L in 24 hours
Urine specific gravity	1.005
Urine osmolality	100 mosm/kg
Urine Na	10 mmol/L

Low specific gravity and low urine osmolality suggest she is unable to concentrate urine.

Her calculated GFR is normal and urine sodium is low. This suggests that renal mechanisms are intact. Polyuria is probably due to psychogenic polydipsia or diabetes insipidus. Patients with psychogenic polydipsia have low sodium in plasma.

The relatively high plasma sodium and low urine Na in the presence of polyuria is diagnostic of diabetes insipidus.

To differentiate central DI from nephrogenic DI water deprivation test is done.

Water Deprivation Test (Miller-Moses Test)

Procedure—Patient is dehydrated by water deprivation for 4–18 hours. Body-weight and urine osmolality are monitored hourly. Normal response is an increase in urine osmolality four to five times greater than plasma. There will be more than 3% reduction in body weight.

Decrease in urine osmolality from normal value or failure of urine osmolality to increase is diagnostic of diabetes insipidus. To differentiate from nephrogenic DI, 5 units of ADH is given subcutaneously and urine osmolality is measured. Normally the increment in osmolaltity is less than 9%. In central DI the increment in urine osmolality is more than 50%.

Water Deprivation Test

Parameter	Value
Decrease in body weight	50 to 48 kg
Urine specific gravity	1.005
Urine osmolality	50 mosm/kg
After ADH infusion	75 mosm/kg

Since, there is increase in urine osmolality after ADH infusion by 50%, diagnosis *is Central diabetes insipidus.*

MANAGEMENT OF HYPERNATREMIA

Management of hypernatremia requires a two-pronged approach:
- Treat the underlying cause
- Correction of hypernatremia

Treat the underlying cause — may involve stopping hypotonic fluid losses, withdraw offending agents like lactulose, diuretics, lithium, treating hyperpyrexia, hyperglycemia, etc.

Correction of the Hypernatremia

Depends on the underlying pathophysiological cause:
- Water and sodium loss
- Pure water loss
- Or excess sodium administration.

Treatment of Euvolemic Hypernatremia (Fig. 5.8)

1. Treat water deficit
2. Prevention of ongoing water losses
3. Vasopressin agonists.

Treatment Guidelines for Hypotonic Fluid Administration

Since hypernatremia = cellular dehydration = ICF volume deficit, ICF volume deficit has to be corrected.

ICF volume is 2/3rd of TBW, i.e. in a 60 kg adult TBW is 36 L and ICF volume is 24 L. ECF volume is 12 liters. Water

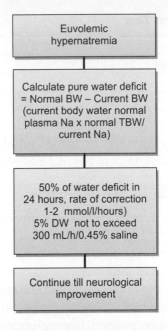

Fig. 5.8: Treatment of euvolemic hypernatremia

distributes into ICF and ECF in the ratio 3:1, when 1 liter of water is infused, 666 mL will enter ICF and 333 mL will be in the ECF.

Type of Fluid

Hypotonic parenteral fluids commonly used are 5% dextrose, half normal saline, or saline diluted to the required Na concentration.

Intravenous administration of distilled water can produce hemolysis, hence is not used.

Route for Correction

Best is oral route, oral intake of water should be encouraged.

Calculation of Deficit

ICF volume deficit can be calculated from plasma sodium.

The short formula used for calculation of ICF volume deficit is

$$\text{"e"}_{normal} \times \text{ICF volume}_{normal} = \text{"e"abnormal} \times \text{ICF volume}_{abnormal}$$

"e" represents effective osmoles = $2 \times Na$

$$\text{ICF volume}_{abnormal} = \frac{\text{"e"normal} \times \text{ICF volume}_{normal}}{\text{"e"abnormal}}$$

ICF volume deficit = ICF volume$_{normal}$ – ICF volume$_{abnormal}$

Example: To calculate the ICF volume deficit in a 60 kg man with a plasma sodium of 160 mmol/L?

ICF volume$_{abnormal}$ = $24 \times 280/320$ = 21 liters.

Hence, ICF volume deficit = 24 – 21 = 3 Liters. *Three liters of water has to be given to reduce the sodium to 140 mmol/L.*

Infusion Rate

The rate of fall in sodium can only be 1 to 2 mmol/L/h, hence the rate of infusion has to be found out, This is given by the formula

{Current Na – (Na – 1)}/current Na × TBW

Here (160-159)/160 × 36 = 3600 mL/160 = 220 mL/h.

- *Replace 50% of water deficit in the first 24 hours.* The remaining water deficit should be corrected in the next 24 hours,
- Measure serum electrolytes, urine sodium and potassium once in 2 hours
- If the sum of urine sodium and potassium is less than the plasma sodium, there is ongoing water loss. Replace ongoing water loss
- If 5% dextrose is used to correct hypernatremia, infusion rate should not exceed 300 mL/h.

The infusion is continued till there is neurological improvement.

Treatment of Hypovolemic Hypernatremia

In hypovolemic hypernatremia there is loss of fluid both from the ECF and ICF, hence the ICF and ECF deficit has to

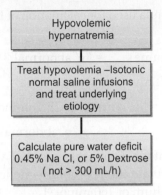

Fig. 5.9: Treatment of hypovolemic hypernatremia

be assessed and corrected. ECF deficit correction—If signs of hypovolemia are present, that should be corrected first with isotonic sodium chloride solutions, Only after correction of hypovolemia, pure water loss has to be calculated and should be corrected (Fig 5.9).

ECF volume deficit is assessed clinically this is shown in Table 5.1.

Treatment of Hypervolemic Hypernatremia

Hypervolemic hypernatremia there is ECF volume expansion and gain of sodium. The common cause is use of hypertonic solutions and first step is stop hypertonic infusions (Fig. 5.10).

- If associated with renal insufficiency, loop diuretics, and or dialysis is to be instituted.
- In case of inadequate thirst, desmopressin is the drug of choice. A synthetic analogue of AVP, desmopressin is available in subcutaneous, intranasal and oral preparations, it can be administered 2–3 times per day. Patients may require hospitalization to establish fluid needs. Frequent electrolyte monitoring is recommended.
- Synthetic vasopressin, the non-hormonal agents chlorpropamide, carbamazepine, clofibrate, thiazides, and indomethacin can be used with caution

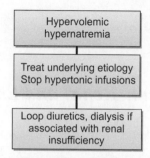

Fig. 5.10: Treatment of hypervolemic hypernatremia

KEY POINTS

- Commonly occurs in neonates, infants and elderly individuals who cannot complain of thirst and cannot drink on their own
- There is net loss of water more than sodium from the body causing hypernatremia
- Hypernatremia" is always a hypertonic state and shifts water from cells.
- Hyperosmolality can result in cellular dehydration and cell shrinkage. The shrinkage of brain can lead to stretching of blood vessels, rupture and hemorrhages.
- Hypernatremia is classified based on ECF volume. Decreased intake of free water is a prerequisite for development of hypernatremia.
- Treatment consists of correction of underlying cause and correction of ICF and ECF deficit. Rate of correction should not be more than 1 mmol/L/h
- Hypotonic fluids are used in correcton
- Over correction can produce cerebral edema.

6

Potassium-Renal and Endocrine Regulation

R Kasi Visweswaran

OVERVIEW

Total body potassium (K) is 50 mmol/kg. In a 70 kg man, it is around 3500 millimoles. 98% of total body K is intracellular and only 2% is extracellular. This difference is achieved by the sodium potassium ATPase pump (Na^+/K^+-ATPase) which is present in all types of animal cells and drives 3 Na^+ out of the cell and transports 2 K^+ into the intracellular compartment. This pump is an active, energy consuming pump that works throughout the life of the cell. The serum level of K^+ is maintained in a narrow range of 3.5–5.0 mmol/L. The atomic weight of K^+ is 39.1 and valency is 1. One mole is molecular weight of any substance in gram dissolved in 1 liter of water. In the case of K^+, 39.1 gm dissolved in 1 liter is 1 mole and 1 millimole is 39.1 mg dissolved 1000 mL. In the case of potassium, since its valency is one, mmol and mEq (milliequivalents) are the same.

Daily dietary intake of K is around 60–100 millimoles. 90% of the daily intake is lost in urine while 10% is excreted through gastrointestinal tract. Potassium homeostasis is maintained by the proportionate increase or decrease in the losses depending on the intake. Maintenance of normal level of K^+ is required for all cellular functions, neuromuscular transmission, cardiac excitability and maintenance of vascular tone.

RENAL HANDLING OF POTASSIUM (FIG. 6.1)

K is completely filtered by the glomerulus. 90% of filtered potassium is reabsorbed in proximal convoluted tubule and loop of Henle. In proximal convoluted tubule, K^+ reabsorption follows water and sodium reabsorption. In the ascending limb of loop of Henle K reabsorption is via the Na - K -2Cl cotransporter.

FACTORS REGULATING K⁺ SECRETION

The K delivered to the distal nephron is constant and the K^+ level in plasma is regulated by increasing or decreasing the secretion of K^+.

As shown in Figure 6.1, Na^+/K^+ ATPase in the basolateral membrane will actively transport K from blood to the cell. This creates a concentration gradient between the cell and the lumen and K will passively enter the lumen. $Na^{+/}K^+$ ATPase will also pump Na out of the cell into the blood. This creates a concentration gradient for Na to move from the lumen to the cell.

FACTORS INCREASING K⁺ SECRETION

1. Mineralocorticoid hormone.
2. High sodium delivery to the collecting duct.

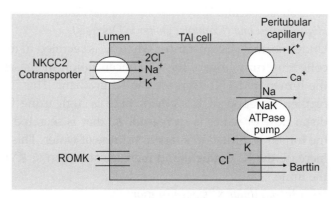

Fig. 6.1: Potassium handling in TAL

3. High urine flow rate caused by osmotic diuretics, protein rich meal, etc.
4. High intracellular K^+ concentration.
5. Low luminal K^+ concentration.
6. Increase in the negativity of lumen by delivery of negatively charged ions to the collecting duct.
7. Increase in the permeability of the luminal membrane.

Mineralocorticoid Hormone

i. Aldosterone is secreted by the zona glomerulosa of adrenal gland. This will bind to the receptor in the cell and stimulate reabsorption of Na^+ from the lumen to the cell. This will make the lumen electronegative and favour K^+ secretion. This is by increasing the open probability of epithelial Na channel.

ii. Increases the $Na/^+K^+ATPase$ activity and increases intracellular K^+ concentration and the gradient.

iii. Increases the permeability of the apical membrane to K^+.

High Sodium Delivery to the Collecting Duct (Example: Diuretics)

Use of loop diuretics will inhibit the reabsorption of Na from loop of Henle. This will increase the delivery of Na^+ to distal tubule and early collecting duct. Na^+ is reabsorbed from the collecting duct lumen. This makes the lumen more electronegative and K^+ is secreted into the lumen.

High Urine Flow (Example: Osmotic Diuresis)

Under normal circumstances when K^+ is secreted in to the collecting duct lumen, the K^+ concentration increases in the lumen and will decrease the K^+ gradient. This limits further secretion of K^+. When there is high urine flow, distal flow of water is increased. K^+ that is secreted into the lumen is diluted in a larger volume of water. This will increase the K^+ gradient and increase secretion of K^+ into the lumen.

High Intracellular K^+ Concentration

POTASSIUM CHANNELS

1. The renal outer medullary K⁺ channel (ROMK) — This is a low conductance and high probability open channel in physiological states.

2. Maxi K⁺ channel is normally quiescent, is active under conditions of increased flow rate. Increased flow bends the primary cilium present in the principal cell. This will increase the intracellular calcium concentration. Maxi channel is calcium activated and will increase secretion of K⁺. The increase in distal flow independent of Na⁺ delivery is shown to activate Na⁺ through the sheer stress (mechanosensitive properties intrinsic to the channel). When a protein rich meal is ingested, this will increase the GFR, increase the distal flow which will activate epithelial Na⁺ channel and also increase intracellular calcium. This also activate maxi channels. Thus, K⁺ secretion is enhanced.

3. With-No-Lysine kinases (WNK) family of kinases — A family of signaling molecules, the WNK (with no K [lysine]) kinases, play a critical role in the regulation of sodium and potassium transport in the distal nephron With-No-Lysine kinases [K] (WNKs) are a recently discovered family of serine/threonine protein kinases. There are four members. Each is coded by a different gene. Mutations in *WNK1* and *WNK4* are linked to *familial hyperkalemic hypertension (FHHt) also known as pseudohypoaldosteronism type II, or Gordon syndrome*. This is characterized by hyperkalemia, metabolic acidosis and hypertension. WNK2, 1% is expressed in all cell lines and tissues.

KS. WNK1 (kidney specific) is expressed only in the kidney and the ratio of KS. WNK 1 to WNK1 is 85% vs 15%.

The L-WNK1 (long form of WNK 1) will increase the endocytosis of ROMK channel and decrease the ROMK in the collecting duct. This will help in K conservation. Potassium

Specific (KS) WNK is a physiological antagonist to the actions of WNK1 and will upregulate ROMK channels and will help in K^+ secretion.

Hyperkalemia often indicates net K^+ gain by the body. However, hypokalemia does not truly reflect the extent of body's potassium loss, since shift of even small quantities of K^+ from intra to extracellular compartment can normalize the serum K^+ level. Intracellular potassium cannot be measured in the clinical laboratory. There is a rough correlation between the degree of hypokalemia and total body potassium deficit. When the serum level is around 3 mmol/L, the body would have lost about 100 millimoles of K^+. When the K^+ is < 2 mmol/L, more than 600 millimoles deficit may be present.

KEY POINTS

- K^+ is predominantly an intracellular ion and hence deficit can be assessed only through the ECF window.
- K^+ losses from the body through urine and GI tract match the intake and K balance is maintained.
- K^+ that is filtered is completely reabsorbed.
- K^+ that is lost in the urine is from the distal tubular secretion.

Hypokalemia

R Kasi Visweswaran

OVERVIEW

Hypokalemia is defined as serum potassium K^+ below 3.5 mmol/L. Patients become symptomatic only when K is less than 3 mmol/L. Potassium (K) is predominantly an intracellular electrolyte. 97–98% of total body potassium is intracellular. It is very difficult to measure intracellular potassium. Changes in ICF potassium is visualized through the tiny window of ECF potassium. ICF Potassium is 150 millimoles/L and ECF potassium is 4.3 millimoles/L. The ratio of ICF to ECF potassium is 35:1. This ratio is always maintained and reduction in potassium from 4 mmol to 3 mmol indicates reduction of ICF potassium around 100 mmol/L. Loss of ICF potassium around 100–400 mmol/L, can result in a high ICF to ECF ratio. Membrane will become hyperpolarized.

HOW DOES THE INTRACELLULAR POTASSIUM CHANGE?

If the ICF has to lose 400 millimoles of potassium, this has to be associated with loss of 400 millimoles of anions from ICF or gain of 400 millimoles of Na^+ or H^+ ions into ICF (Fig. 7.1).

Why Recognize Hypokalemia?

Hypokalemia can affect all systems. The clinical consequences are described below.

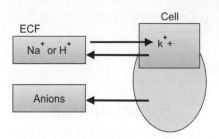

Fig. 7.1: Intracellular potassium shift

Hyperglycemia is due to impaired insulin release and decreased sensitivity to insulin.

Cardiovascular system can cause cardiac arrhythmias and sudden death. Predisposing factors are congestive heart failure, underlying ischemic heart disease/acute myocardial ischemia, aggressive therapy for hyperglycemia as in diabetic ketoacidosis, digitalis therapy, Conn syndrome, etc. Hypokalemia is a risk factor for hypertension and end organ damage.

Hypokalemia precipitates **hepatic encephalopathy** in patients with liver disease.

Hypokalemia induces resistance to the action of ADH and cause nephrogenic diabetes insipidus.

Hyperglycemia is due to impaired insulin release and decreased sensitivity to insulin. Hyperglycemia can cause endothelial cell dysfunction. Increased risk of overt athero-sclerosis is due to altered lipid metabolism.

Can alter vascular reactivity, resulting in enhanced vasoconstriction and impaired relaxation with clinical sequelae. Ischemic central nervous system events or rhabdomyolysis.

Produces muscle weakness, depression of the deep-tendon reflexes, and flaccid paralysis.

Decreases gut motility, leading to or exacerbating paralytic ileus.

Hypokalemia is associated with high mortality in stress conditions such as myocardial infarction, septic shock, diabetic ketoacidosis.

Clinical Approach to Hypokalemia

If potassium value is low and the clinical scenario does not explain hypokalemia, Pseudohypokalemia (spurious) should be excluded.

Pseudohypokalemia (Spurious hypokalemia) — This is an in vitro phenomenon and occurs when blood sample is stored especially in high ambient temperature. In patients, with leukemia and high leucocyte counts, K^+ may be taken up into the abnormal WBCs (in vitro) after collection of blood sample. This is known as pseudohypokalemia and when the serum K^+ is unexpectedly low, the blood count results must be reviewed. This in vitro phenomenon can be prevented by rapid separation of the sample and storing serum sample at 4°C. When there is no obvious cause for hypokalemia, Pseudohypokalemia should be excluded by analyzing the sample immediately after collection.

Case History 1

A Seven-year-old child is admitted with pneumonia and leukocytosis.
Investigations

Parameter in plasma/blood	
Total count	*25000/cmm.*
FBS	85 mg%
Urea	26 mg%
Creatinine	1.2 mg%
Na	140 mmol/L
K	3 mmol/L

The significant biochemical abnormality in this child was a plasma potassium of 3 mmol/L. There was no known cause for hypokalemia. When potassium estimation was repeated immediately after collection it showed normal value. Here hypokalemia was pseudo or spurious hypokalemia.

True hypokalemia can be due to redistribution of potassium and or reduction in total body potassium (Fig. 7.2).

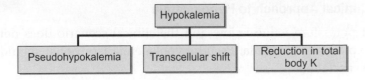

Fig. 7.2: Causes of hypokalemia

Hypokalemia Due to Redistribution (Fig. 7.4)

More than 98% of body's K^+ is intracellular and the movement of potassium between the ICF and ECF compartment is regulated by numerous factors. The plasma level of K^+ can decrease due to insulin, aldosterone, β_2 adrenergic agonists, alkalosis or cellular (muscle) injury.

- Hormones and drugs
- Hypokalemic periodic paralysis
- Delirium tremens
- Barium poisoning
- Hyperthyroidism
- Metabolic alkalosis.

Hormones and Drugs

Catecholamines

Catecholamines are increased in response to stress, hypoglycemia, exercise and hypotension. This can cause shift of K^+ into the cell. This action is mediated through a rise in cyclic AMP leading to phosphorylation and activation of Na^+/K^+-ATPase. The resting membrane potential (RMP) is made more negative.

β_2-adrenergic Agonists and Theophylline

β_2-adrenergic agonists and theophylline contained in bronchodilators, decongestants and tocolytics also induce hypokalemia. Mechanism is same as catecholamine induced K shift into cell. With the usual dose, plasma K falls by 0.2–0.3 millimoles/L.

Overdose of these group of drugs can reduce K by 0.5–2 mmol/L.

Insulin

Insulin makes RMP more negative. There is increased electroneutral entry of Na via $Na^+ - H^+$ antiporter. The increased Na^+ in cell stimulates the electrogenic Na^+/K^+-ATPase in basolateral membrane. There is increased accumulation of anions like phosphate esters. Exit of Na and accumulation of anions especially makes RMP more negative and results in hyperpolarization. This is seen when massive doses of insulin is used in the treatment of diabetic ketoacidosis.

Hypokalemic Periodic Paralysis

It is a rare hereditary disease due to mutation in cell membrane dihydropyridine sensitive calcium channel. Severe hypokalemia is triggered by heavy carbohydrate meal, sodium intake or exercise. Hypokalemia leads to development of flaccid paralysis and respiratory failure due to hypoventilation. With correction of K^+ deficiency and ventilatory support when indicated the paralysis resolves dramatically (Fig. 7.3).

Hyperthyroidism leads to hypokalemia by stimulating Na+/K+-ATPase activity. Hypokalemic periodic paralysis occurs in conjunction with hyperthyroidism. If family history is negative in a patient who presents with hypokalemia and periodic paralysis, hyperthyroidism should be excluded (Fig. 7.3).

Delirium Tremens

Increased endogenous β adrenergic stimulation leads to hypokalemia.

Barium Poisoning

Blocks the exit of K^+ from the cell leading to hypokalemia.

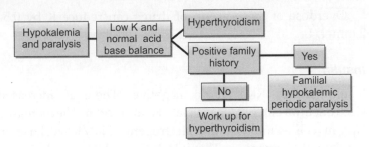

Fig. 7.3: Hypokalemia and muscle paralysis

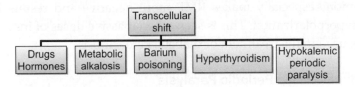

Fig. 7.4: Causes of transcellular shift of potassium

Metabolic Alkalosis

Excess bicarbonate is filtered into the lumen. H^+ exits from the cell via $Na^+ H^+$ antiporter. Cell becomes more positive, stimulates $Na^+/K^+ATPase$ and 3 Na exchanges with 2 potassium. RMP becomes more negative, in hyperpolarized state.

Case History 2

A 50-year-old lady with history of chronic obstructive pulmonary disease was admitted with exacerbation of dyspnea. She was managed with β adrenergic agonists. She presented with muscular weakness.

Investigations are as follows.

Blood/serum

RBS	104 mg%
Urea	32 mg%
Creatinine	1.3 mg%
Na	138 mmol/L
K	3.1 mmol/L

Patient has normal GFR with low potassium

ABG Values	
pH	7.32
pCO$_2$	50 mm Hg
PaO$_2$	78 mmHg
HCO$_3$	25 mmol/L
O$_2$sat	90%

Diagnosis: Hypokalemia and respiratory acidosis

What is the cause of hypokalemia? Hypokalemic in this patient is due to transcellular shift of K+ from ECF to ICF caused by β agonists.

Hypokalemia can result in respiratory muscle fatigue, and exacerbate respiratory acidosis. Withdrawal of β$_2$ adrenergic agonists will help to correct hypokalemia and also improve muscle weakness.

APPROACH TO TRUE HYPOKALEMIA

True hypokalemia is associated with reduction in total body potassium. Reduction in total body K$^+$ can be due to renal or extrarenal losses. Most common cause for true hypokalemia is increased loss of K in urine (Fig. 7.5).

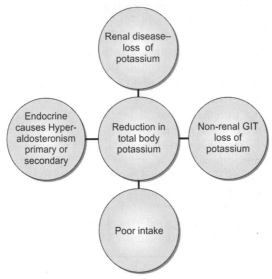

Fig. 7.5: Causes for the reduction in total body potassium

Case History 3

A 12-year-old child is admitted with flaccid paralysis following watery diarrhea. There is no history of poor dietary intake, renal disease, drug intake or other significant past illness

Investigations

Parameter in plasma/blood

Total count	5000/cmm.
FBS	85 mg%
Urea	46 mg%
Creatinine	1.2 mg%
Na	135 mmol/L
K	2.3 mmol/L
Cl	114 mmol/L

Patient has elevated plasma urea, normal creatinine and low potassium. The low potassium is responsible for flaccid paralysis.

Hypokalemia is as a result of reduction in total body potassium

Loss of potassium can be through renal loss or extrarenal loss.

To find out whether the loss is renal or extrarenal, 24 hours urinary potassium loss has to be estimated.

This can be measured after collecting urine for 24 hours.

A simple formula can also be used to extrapolate potassium in random sample to 24 hour urine loss.

24 hour urine potassium = (urine K in mmol/L ÷ urine creatinine in millimoles) × anticipated creatinine excretion in 24 hours

(0.2 × wt: in kg for males and 0.17 × wt: in kg for females).

In patients, with normal GFR, creatinine secretion is constant at 17 mg/kg in females and 20 mg/kg in 24 hours, Conversion formula for creatinine to micromoles is 1 mg = 88 micromoles.

In a 50 kg man if K is of 20 mmol/L and Cr: is 18 miilimoles, in random urine sample

24 hours urinary K = 20/18 × (0.2 × 50) = 11 millimoles).

If 24 hours urinary potassium is < 20 mmol/L, loss is extrarenal and if > 20 mmol/L loss is renal.

The following steps are used to evaluate true hypokalemia.

Step 1: Measure urinary potassium

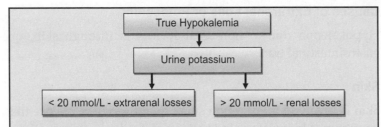

In this patient 24 hour, urinary potassium is 11 millimoles. Therefore, hypokalemia is due to loss of potassium through extrarenal route.
Step 2: To find out the cause of extra renal loss, correlate with ABG. The causes of extra renal potassium loss can be diagnosed by ABG status. The causes associated with metabolic acidosis, metabolic alkalosia and variable pH is shown in Figure 7.6

Metabolic acidosis indicates GI loss, normal pH is a clue to decreased intake of potassium in diet, or use of laxatives. Metabolic alkalosis can be seen in villous adenoma, laxative use, and congenital chloridorrhea

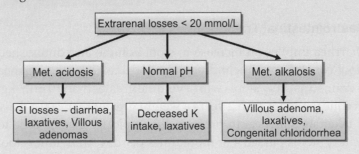

Fig. 7.6: Causes for hypokalemia based on ABG status

Next step is to Assess ABG status

ABG values in this patient

pH	7.26
PCO₂	27 mm Hg
PaO₂	98 mm Hg
HCO₃	12 mmol/L
O₂sat	98%

This patient has metabolic acidosis. Patient has low urinary K with metabolic acidosis. This suggests diarrhea as the cause of hypokalemia.

Causes of Extrarenal Loss of Potassium

Hypokalemia due to non-renal K^+ loss is through skin, or gastrointestinal tract.

Skin

Skin is involved in excretion small quantities of K^+, hence the quantum of loss from skin is minimal. To decrease potassium by 1 mmol, there should be at least 100 millimoles loss of K. As shown, 1 liter of sweat contains only 5 millimoles of potassium, 20 liters of sweat should be lost and this is extremely rare.

Composition of sweat is shown below.

Na	40 mmol/L
K	5 mmol/L
Cl	50 mmol/L

Gastrointestinal Tract

Diarrhea implies an increase in stool volume and diminished stool consistency. In children younger than 2 years, diarrhea is defined as daily stools with a volume greater than 10 mL/kg. In children older than 2 years a weight greater than 200 g daily is taken as diarrhea. In practice, this typically means loose to watery stools passed 4 or more times per day. Individual stool patterns vary widely; for example, breastfeeding children may normally have 5–6 stools per day.

Composition of secretions from ileum and colon is shown below.

Secretion	Ileum	Colon
Volume/24 h	3000	
Na mmol/L	140	60
K mmol/L	5	30
Cl mmol/L	104	40
HCO$_3$ mmol/L	30	0

Around 30 mmol/L of potassium K^+ is secreted into the colon. In colonic diarrheas, chronic laxative abuse, and repeated enemas, large amount of K is lost and this excessive K^+ loss through large bowel can cause hypokalemia. The small intestine secretion of potassium is very low only 5 mmol/L. So Patients with high output jejunal or ileostomies do not develop hypokalemia

Decreased Dietary Intake

If renal function is normal and there is no loss of potassium or shift of potassium from ECF into ICF, decreased intake alone will not cause hypokalemia.

It is very rarely seen in elderly patients who are unable to chew or swallow and in patients receiving total parenteral nutrition for prolonged periods without potassium supplementation. Alcoholic patients on "fruit of vine" diet, elderly patients on "Tea-toast" diet and patients with anorexia nervosa can develop hypokalemia due to decreased dietary intake of potassium. Geophagia is a condition where patients ingest large amount of clay. This will bind potassium secreted in the GI tract and potassium will not be available for absorption. In conditions, associated with increased body needs as in recovery from meagaloblastic anemia, hyperalimentation state, and transfusion with frozen erythrocytes, hypokalemia may ensue. In these patients arterial pH is normal.

Villous Adenomas

Villous adenomas (rare cause of diarrhea) this is a rare cause of diarrhea more often associated with larger adenomas and more severe degrees of dysplasia. These adenomas occur more frequently in the rectum and rectosigmoid. Metabolic acidosis and metabolic alkalosis are known to occur in villous adenomas.

Hypokalemia due to secretion of large volume of mucin rich in potassium may contribute to metabolic alkalosis. Loss of colonic secretions that are rich in bicarbonate cause metabolic acidosis.

Congenital Chloridorrhea

Congenital chloridorrhea is a rare form of severe secretory diarrhea that is inherited as an autosomal recessive trait. Mutations in the down-regulated adenoma gene result in defective function of the chloride/bicarbonate exchange in the colon and ileum, leading to increased secretion of chloride and reabsorption of bicarbonate. This may lead to metabolic alkalosis.

CAUSES OF RENAL LOSS OF POTASSIUM

Renal loss is the most common cause for true hypokalemia.

Case History 4

A 75-five-year old lady with history of hypertension is admitted with complete heart block. She developed pulmonary edema and her BP was 120/80 mm Hg
Investigations are as follows.

Variables in blood/plasma	Day 1	Day 3
RBS	209 mg%	114 mg%
Urea	35 mg%	34 mg%
Creatinine	1.1 mg%	1.3 mg%
Na^+	139 mmol /L	134 mmol/L
K^+	4.7 mmol/L	3 mmol/L
Cl^-	98 mmol/L	90 mmol/L
HCO_3	20.1 mmol/L	21.5 mmol/L

Patient developed hypokalemia on the third day of admission following correction of hyperglycemia with insulin and administration of orciprenaline and frusemide.
Hypokalemia can be due to two causes in this patient.
1. Due to shift of K from ECF to ICF by orciprenaline and insulin
2 . Frusemide can produce increased loss of potassium in urine.

As discussed earlier the first step is to estimate urine K, and other electrolytes Na, and chloride.

Urine electrolytes	Day 3
Na	46 mmol/L
K	52 mmol/L
Cl⁻	81 mmol/L

Patient has normal creatinine, mild hyponatremia, with urinary loss of Na, hypokalemia with urinary loss of K > 20 mmol/L and urine chloride > 20 mmol/L indicating increased loss of K in urine.

Second step is to find out the acid base status. The causes of renal potassium loss can be diagnosed by ABG status.The causes associated with metabolic acidosis, metabolic alkalosis and variable pH is shown in Figure 7.7.

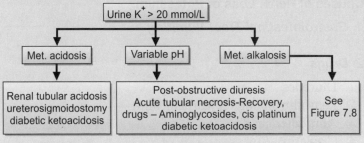

Fig. 7.7: Causes of hypokalemia with renal loss based on ABG

ABG status of the patient

Parameter	Day 3
pH	7.52
pCO_2	35 mm Hg
HCO_3	30 mmol/L
PaO_2	144 mm Hg (FiO_2-28%)

ABG shows metabolic alkalosis and respiratory alkalosis

Step 3: Proceed as in metabolic alkalosis, estimate urine chloride. Urine chloride in this patient is 80 mmol/L indicating failure to conserve chloride.

In this patient, Hypokalemia, is due to transcellular shift caused by orciprenaline and Insulin. There is also renal loss of potassium due to frusemide.

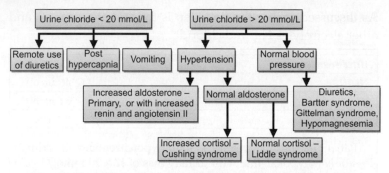

Fig. 7.8: Hypokalemia with metabolic alkalosis- based on urine chloride

Approach to hypokalemia with metabolic alkalosis-estimate urine chloride (Fig. 7.8).

Causes of Renal Loss of Potassium

1. Gastrointestinal Tract-Vomiting

2. Drugs

1. Diuretics
2. Penicillin analogues (carbenicillin)
3. Amphotericin B
4. Cisplatin
5. Aminoglycosides
6. Toluene.

3. Endogenous Hormones Mineralocorticoid Excess

1. Primary hyperaldosteronism
2. Congenital adrenal hyperplasia
3. Glucocorticoid responsive aldosteronism
4. High dose glucocorticoids.

4. Diuresis (Polyuria due to any cause)

1. Resolving stage of acute kidney injury
2. Postobstructive diuresis
3. Partial ureteric obstruction
4. Renal tubular acidosis (RTA).

5. Magnesium depletion

6. Bicarbonaturia

7. Intrinsic renal tubular potassium transport abnormalities

1. Bartter syndrome
2. Gitelman syndrome
3. Liddle syndrome
4. Syndrome of apparent mineralocorticoid excess
5. Glucocorticoid remediable aldosteronism.

Gastrointestinal Tract

Vomiting

There is loss of gastric juice alone in vomiting due conditions like pyloric stenosis or continuous nasogastric aspiration Gastric juice contains only 10mmol/L Vomiting or continuous nasogastric aspiration may result in loss of only 5-8 millimoles/L of K$^+$ in the drained fluid. So to reduce ECF potassium by 1mmol/L, total K loss should be at least 100 moles – loss of gastric juice should be around 10 L. Hypokalemia in these patients is due to the loss of H$^+$ ions, development of metabolic alkalosis and secondary hyperaldosteronism which results in increased urinary K$^+$ loss. Hypokalemia in vomiting is mainly due to loss of K in urine.

Drugs

Diuretics

Use of thiazide or loop diuretics result in hypokalemia and is related to the dose and duration of therapy. Hypokalemia is more common when infusion of diuretic is used.

Mechanisms by which thiazide and loop diuretics Cause Hypokalemia

i. **By increasing distal delivery of Na:** These diuretics inhibit sodium reabsorption resulting in *Increased delivery of sodium* *to the collecting ducts.* The Na/K exchanger actively exchange more Na for K resulting in K loss. The increased delivery of K to the collecting ducts facilitates the exchange of K for H by the H^+/K^+ exchangers on the intercalated alpha cells, resulting in loss of H^+ leading to the development of metabolic alkalosis).

ii. By activation of renin-angiotensin- aldosterone system by the diuretic induced hypovolemia: Physiological response to hypovolemia is activation of RAAS and release of aldosterone. This stimulates the Na^+/K^+ exchanger, resulting in further loss of potassium. Diuretics increase the flow rate in the nephron. So the luminal fluid K is diluted resulting in greater gradient between the cell and lumen. Potassium diffuse through many potassium channels, such as ROMK into the lumen. ROMK is not an exchanger system, they allow facilitated diffusion along a concentration gradient.

Penicillin Analogues

Presence of excess of unabsorbable anions in the lumen of the distal tubule as in carbenicillin use results in diffusion of K^+ ion into the tubular lumen to neutralize the anionic charge.

Amphotericin B

Increases K^+ secretion into the collecting duct and results in hypokalemia.

Cisplatin

Cisplatin causes hypomagnesemia and hypokalemia.

Aminoglycosides

Toluene

Exposure to toluene, by sniffing toluene containing glues lead to distal renal tubular acidosis, renal K^+ wasting and hypokalemia.

Endogenous Hormones

Most conditions associated with mineralocorticoid excess particularly aldosterone cause hypokalemia by increasing the renal potassium excretion and promoting intracellular shift of potassium. Since glucocorticoid hormones also activate mineralocorticoid receptors, high dose glucocorticoids also cause hypokalemia. Genetic defects like glucocorticoid remediable aldosteronism and congenital adrenal hyperplasia are associated with excessive aldosterene production and hypokalemia.

Diuresis (Polyuria Due to Any Cause)

Most polyuric conditions like recovering stage of acute kidney injury (earlier called diuretic phase of acute renal failure), postobstructive diuresis, polyuria following relief of acute urinary obstruction, partial urinary obstruction which produces polyuria due to functional defects in the collecting tubule function or renal tubular acidification defects like renal tubular acidosis (except type IV renal tubular acidosis which causes hyperkalemia) cause hypokalemia. These conditions are commonly encountered in day to day practice and awareness is important for early recognition and prompt correction of this electrolyte abnormality.

Magnesium Depletion

This is closely linked to hypokalemia. Magnesium depletion inhibits renal tubular ability to reabsorb K^+. Mg^{++} depletion occurs in diuretic, aminoglycoside or cisplatin induced hypokalemia. Hypokalemia cannot be corrected unless Mg^{++} deficiency is corrected simultaneously. Therefore, whenever hypokalemia cannot be corrected by adequate K^+ supplements, associated Mg^{++} deficiency should be suspected.

Bicarbonaturia

Bicarbonaturia may occur in patients with metabolic alkalosis, distal renal tubular acidosis or during treatment of proximal renal tubular acidosis. When tubular bicarbonate delivery is increased, K^+ secretion occurs resulting in hypokalemia.

INTRINSIC RENAL TUBULAR POTASSIUM TRANSPORT ABNORMALITIES

Three rare inherited syndromes due to intrinsic renal potassium transport defects leading to hypokalemia and metabolic alkalosis are Bartter syndrome, Gitelman's syndrome and Liddle's syndrome.

Although they are rare, the pathogenesis and pathophysiology is interesting and these syndromes will be discussed in some detail.

In the TAL (thick ascending limb), as in all other cells, the active Na^+/K^+-ATPase in the basolateral membrane keeps the Na^+ out of the cell while increasing the intracellular K^+. The K^+ diffuses into the low potassium containing tubular fluid through the Renal Outer Medullary potassium channel (ROMK) ROMK channel is an ATP sensitive channel and helps to move potassium to the lumen. Sodium and chloride are already present in the lumen here. These three are substrates important for efficient working of sodium, potassium, 2 chloride $(NaKCl_2)$ cotransporter system from the lumen to the cell. Thus reabsorption of Na and chloride occurs in this segment. The basolateral membrane of the cell has K^+ and Cl^- cotransporter which enable K^+ and Cl^- to come to the peritubular capillary. The K^+ gets back into the cell through Na^+/K^+-ATPase. The chloride can also move through the basolateral chloride channel called ClC-Kb. A protein in the beta subunit of the channel called Barttin is essential for the adequate working of this channel. In the TAL, the $NaKCl_2$ cotransporter is sensitive to frusemide (Fig. 7.9).

The distal segment of the DCT and the upper collecting duct has a transporter that reabsorbs about 1–2% of filtered sodium in exchange for potassium and hydrogen ion, which are excreted into the urine. In the distal convoluted

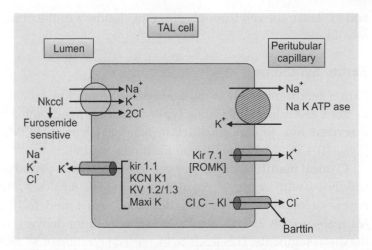

Fig. 7.9: Potassium handling in TAL

NKCCl. Na /K/2Cl co transporter; Kir1.1. inward rectifying channel (ROMK); KV 1.2,1.3. voltage gated K channel, KCN K 1- two pore K channel; Maxi K. voltage and Ca gated K channel; Cl C. Kb basolateral chloride channel containing Bartin

tubule. K$^+$ is secreted by the principal cells in the cortical and outer medullary collecting tubule and the papillary (or inner medullary) collecting duct. Na$^+$ and Cl$^-$ enter the cell from the tubular lumen through a thiazide sensitive Na$^+$Cl$^-$ cotransporter (NCCT). Na$^+$ Cl$^-$ leave the cell to the peritubular side through the action of Na$^+$/K$^+$-ATPase and chloride channel respectively. Calcium enters the cell from the tubular lumen through calcium channels and moves to the peritubular capillary blood through the Na$^+$-Ca$^+$ exchanger in the basolateral membrane. On the luminal side, epithelial sodium channel (ENaC) transports Na$^+$ from the lumen to the cell and is moved out into peritubular capillary by the Na/K-ATPase. This channel is sensitive to amiloride. Both ENaC and Na$^+$/K$^+$-ATPase are stimulated by aldosterone. The action of aldosterone is mediated through mineralocorticoid receptor. Cortisol also stimulates the mineralocorticoid receptor in this segment. Thus, sodium reabsorption is increased and K$^+$

and H⁺ leave the cell through different channels in the apical membrane.

Bartter Syndrome

Bartter syndrome is due to mutation of cell membrane proteins in thick ascending limb. Four types of Bartter syndrome are described due to abnormalities in $NaKCl_2$ (Type I), ROMK (Type II), CIC- Kb (Type III) and Barttin (Type 1V).

Clinical manifestations: may present in perinatal period or childhood with severe hypokalemia, metabolic alkalosis and normal or low blood pressure. As discussed earlier the defective Na reabsorption in TAL results in higher sodium delivery to the distal segments. This leads to increased secretion of K⁺ and H⁺ ions wasting K⁺ and H⁺ leading to severe hypokalemia and metabolic alkalosis. The urinary excretion of K⁺ and Cl⁻ may be high, depending on the age of onset and severity.

Management: Bartter's syndrome is managed with saline infusions, potassium supplementation and magnesium supplementation if necessary. ACE inhibitors are beneficial and therapy is lifelong.

With appropriate therapy some children improve and grow to adulthood. Interstitial disease may progress and may lead to progressive renal failure

Gitelman's Syndrome

This is an autosomal recessive condition and is due to abnormal gene for NCCT which results in inactivation of thiazide sensitive NCCT. The high Na⁺ in distal tubule leads to increased K⁺ and H⁺ excretion.

This syndrome is also associated with hypokalemia, metabolic alkalosis and increased excretion of chloride in urine. The blood pressure is often normal, long term magnesium and potassium supplementation offers partial symptomatic relief and the prognosis is good (Fig. 7.10).

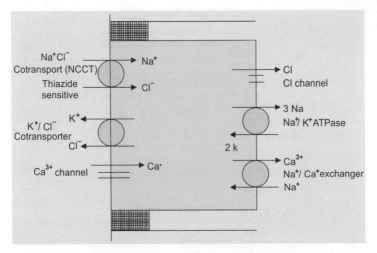

Fig. 7.10: Potassium handling in distal tubule

Liddle's Syndrome (Pseudohyperaldosteronism)

Liddle's syndrome is inherited as autosomal dominant condition and is due to mutation in the ENaC in the collecting duct. The mutation causes persistence of ENaC in the apical membrane therefore ENaC channels are increased in number. This leads to increased sodium reabsorption, hypertension, hypokalemia and metabolic alkalosis. Although these patients have features of primary hyperaldosteronism, the serum aldosterone and renin levels are lower and the hypokalemia does not respond to aldosterone antagonists. Therapy is mainly **sodium** restriction and potassium supplementation (Fig. 7.11).

CLINICAL MANIFESTATIONS OF HYPOKALEMIA

Milder forms of hypokalemia are asymptomatic. Severe hypokalemia is associated with acute onset of symptoms relating to cardiovascular and neuromuscular systems.

In the cardiovascular system, hypokalemia predisposes to cardiac arrhythmias and digitalis toxicity. In patients with

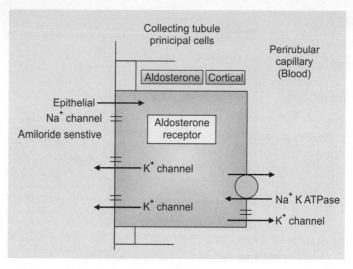

Fig. 7.11: Potassium handling in distal tubule and early collecting duct

underlying cardiac disease or in those on digitalis, even minimal decrease in serum or total body K⁺ may cause supra ventricular or ventricular arrhythmias. The characteristic ECG abnormalities include 'U' waves, QT prolongation and ST depression. Involvement of smooth muscles in the GIT results in constipation and paralytic ileus. In the urinary system, urinary retention may occur. Patients may develop skeletal muscle weakness, cramps is an early manifestation, tetany, muscle necrosis and rhabdomyolysis or even flaccid paralysis may occur.

Chronic manifestations of hypokalemia are more manifested in endocrine and renal systems. Endocrine manifestations are Carbohydrate intolerance, diabetes mellitus or growth retardation in children.

Decrease in glomerular filtration rate, increased ammoniagenesis, polyuria with nephrogenic diabetes insipidus, chloride sensitive metabolic alkalosis, are the functional sequelae. Long standing hypokalemia may produce tubular vacuolation, interstitial nephritis or cyst formation.

TREATMENT OF HYPOKALEMIA

The goal of pharmacotherapy is to correct deficiency, prevent complications, and reduce morbidity.

Guidelines for Correction of Hypokalemia

Aims:

1. To decrease potassium losses
2. To replenish potassium stores,
3. Find out whether any potential for toxicity from correction and
4. Determine the cause to prevent future episodes.

First Step is to Decrease Potassium Loss

- Discontinue diuretics/laxatives.
- Use potassium-sparing diuretics if diuretic therapy is required in disease states like severe heart failure.
- Treat diarrhea or vomiting.
- Use H_2 blockers to decrease nasogastric suction losses.
- Control hyperglycemia.
- In patients with low intake or increased demands, increase intake

Second Step is to Replete Potassium Loss

For every decrease in serum potassium of 1 mmol/L, the total body potassium deficit is approximately 100–300 mmol. Other factors including alkalosis, drugs and hormones cause shift of K^+ to ICF and decrease ECF potassium. With the correction of underlying abnormalities K may shift from ICF to ECF. Therefore only 1/4th of the calculated whole body deficit is corrected at a time and the condition reevaluated frequently by serum potassium monitoring.

The following table gives the approximate whole body K^+ deficit for a given serum K^+ level, assuming pH is normal.

Whole body K^+ deficit for a given serum K^+ level at pH of 7.4

Serum K level	Approximate body K⁺ deficit
3 mmol/L	300 mmol
2 mmol/L	400–600 mmol
< 2 mmol/L	> 600 mmol

This calculation could either over estimate or under estimate the true potassium deficit depending on other factors that influence serum K, The risk to develop hyperkalemia is minimal with oral potassium supplements. Oral potassium replacement should be preferred over parenteral potassium supplementation.

Potassium can be replaced as dietary supplements and solutions containing potassium. Potassium is absorbed readily. Relatively large doses can be given safely. Some individuals develop nausea or even gastrointestinal ulceration when concentrated enteral potassium formulations are given. **Potassium chloride** is available as Potassium chloride solution. 15 mL contains 20 mmol of K.

One tablet provides 8 mmoles of K^+. The usual oral dose is 20 mmoles 3–4 times a day. In severe cases, it can be increased to 40 mmoles thrice daily. Since oral K^+ supplements cause gastric irritation, it is advisable to dilute the solution or use the tablet in a glass of water. **Potassium citrate** is used for patients who form calcium stones or has severe metabolic acidosis.

The indications for aggressive correction of hypokalemia to a level of 3.5 mmoles/L are

- Hypokalemic periodic paralysis
- Patient requiring emergency surgery
- Acute myocardial infarction with life-threatening arrhythmia
- Diabetic ketoacidosis
- Non-ketotic diabetic coma.

Contraindications for Aggressive Correction

- Patients with anuria/oliguria
- Patients on potassium sparing diuretics, ACE inhibitiors
- Patients with digitalis toxicity.

Intravenous potassium - To tide over emergency, I/V potassium chloride infusion may be given perenterally under ECG monitoring. Bolus infusions and rapid infusion may precipitate fatal cardiac arrhythmia and should not be given.

Potassium chloride is available as 7.5% solution in 10 mL ampoules, One mL contains 2 mmoles of K^+. This potassium chloride, can be highly irritating to veins, can precipitate sudden death. It should be administered only as infusions.

For dilution, Potassium chloride can be added to 20% mannitol (if GFR is normal) or normal saline. Solution should be shaken well before use. *Two ampoules of KCl diluted in 500 mL normal saline given at 25 drops/min provides 8 mmol/L/h.* Continuous ECG monitoring and frequent K^+ level estimation are mandatory. Once the emergency is tided over, correction must be gentle and spread over many days.

5% dextrose and glucose-containing parenteral fluids should be avoided as a diluent since it can aggravate hypokalemia by insulin induced shift to ICF.

Potassium infusions can be given only in relatively small doses, generally 10 mmol/h.

It is advisable not to exceed 10–20 mmol/h, 240 mmol/ day and a concentration of 40 mmol/L. (1 ampoule of KCl in 500 mL of normal saline = 20 mmoles).

Under close cardiac supervision in emergency circumstances, up to a maximum of 40 mmol/h can be administered through a central line.

Commonly used potassium containing IV fluids are

Solution	K concentration
Ringer's lactate	4 mmol/L
Isolyte G	17 mmol/L
Isolyte M	35. mmol/L

- Oral and parenteral potassium can be used simultaneously with close monitoring of K level.

Calculation of Requirement of Potassium

For finding out the K deficit, the volume and concentration of K in the fluid lost should be taken into consideration.

- In conditions like diarrhea, where acidosis and hypokalemia coexist, *hypokalemia should be corrected first.*

Otherwise, correction of acidosis or development of alkalosis can worsen hypokalemia by shift of potassium into the cells. **Hypomagnesemia should also be corrected along with hypokalemia.**

- **Tailor treatment to the individual patient.** For example, if diuretics cannot be discontinued due to an underlying disorder such as congestive heart failure, institute potassium sparing therapies, -low sodium diet, potassium sparing diuretics, ACE inhibitors and angiotensin receptor blockers. The low-sodium diet and potassium-sparing diuretics limit the amount of sodium reabsorbed at the cortical collecting tubule, thus limiting the amount of potassium secreted. ACE inhibitors and angiotensin receptor blockers inhibit the release of aldosterone, thus blocking the kaliuretic effects of that hormone. Naturally occurring potassium rich food such as fruit juice, tender coconut water, dry fruits and some salt substitutes can also be used as oral K^+ supplements. Among the IV fluids, Ringer's lactate contains 4 millimoles/L Isolyte G-17 millimoles/L and isolyte M 35 mmol/L. Rarely, simultaneous use of K^+ sparing diuretics, ACE inhibitors and dietary sodium restrictions are essential with oral K^+ supplements to correct hypokalemia. In any situation, when hypokalemia does not respond well to correction, simultaneous Mg^{++} deficiency is looked for and corrected.

KEY POINTS

- Confronted with low potassium value, confirm this is true hypokalemia.
- In true hypokalemia, find out the route of loss by estimating urinary potassium.

- Correlate with ABG status and find out the probable cause.
- Mild hypokalemia, can be corrected by withdrawing medications if any, supplementing potassium rich diet.
- Moderate hypokalemia can be corrected by oral potassium chloride/or citrate.
- Severe hypokalemia can be corrected by parenteral potassium chloride by strictly following the guidelines.

Hyperkalemia

R Kasi Visweswaran

OVERVIEW AND RISK FACTORS

Hyperkalemia is a medical emergency. It is defined as serum potassium (K^+) > 5.5 mmol/L. It is rare in healthy general population. Certain groups are at higher risk for hyperkalemia. The common risk factors are:

1. *Military recruits, drug abusers, and patients with sickle cell trait* because they have a high risk for acute rhabdomyolysis. There is a high incidence in males.

2. *Men are at increased risk* due to the high muscle mass. An underlying hormonal predisposition has also been suggested. Exact reason is not known.

3. *Premature infants* are at high risk probably due to renal immaturity and reduction in GFR.

4. *Elderly patients (older than 60 years) are at high risk* because there is decline in renal blood flow and decline in GFR due to ageing process. There is decrease in renin activity and aldosterone levels resulting in reduced ability of distal nephron to secrete potassium ions.

5. *Patients on angiotensin converting enzyme inhibitors* (ACEIs), angiotensin receptor blockers (ARBs), β blockers, Potassium sparing diuretics or aldosterone receptor blockers may develop hyperkalemia.

6. Heparin can reduce aldosterone and result in hyperkalemia in elderly bedridden patients who are on heparin for prevention of DVT,
7. Patients with diabetes mellitus are at high risk due to the following factors:
   a. Diabetic diet is rich in potassium.
   b. There is relative deficiency of insulin or resistance to the action of insulin resulting in inability to shift K from ECF to ICF.
   c. Angiotensin converting enzyme inhibitors (ACEIs), Angiotensin receptor blockers (ARBs) used for prevention of diabetic nephropathy can precipitate hyperkalemia. Risk factors for hyperkalemia in patients on ACEIs, ARBs therapy are *impaired GFR, advanced age, diabetes mellitus with type IV RTA, congestive cardiac failure, longer duration of treatment with ACEIs and ARBs, co prescription with betablockers, potassium sparing diuretics, aldosterone receptor blockers.*
   d. Peripheral vascular disease.
   e. Hyporeninemic hypoaldosteronism (type IV RTA) in chronic tubulo interstitial nephritis can cause hyperkalemia.

WHY TO RECOGNIZE HYPERKALEMIA?

This is considered a "silent killer". Hyperkalemia is not associated with specific symptoms or clinical signs. The ECG changes or serum levels may point to the diagnosis, Vague muscle weakness with hyporeflexia and paralysis of limb and trunk muscles occur in severe cases. Rarely, patients present with hyperkalemic periodic paralysis. Hyperkalemia is an independent risk factor for death. Very high mortality (28%) is reported in patients with K > 7 mmol/L because of cardiac arrhythmias culminating in cardiac arrest.

Therefore, hyperkalemia is a potentially fatal condition. Prompt detection and treatment is rewarding. There is no strict correlation between the degree of hyperkalemia and cardiac abnormalities. The rate of development of hyperkalemia is as important as degree of hyperkalemia. The kidneys are capable of elimination of excessive potassium till the stage of advanced renal failure (stage IV and V of CKD). Hence persistent hyperkalemia is usually seen only in advanced renal failure. If GFR is 30 ml/mt and serum K is high, low aldosterone bioactivity or reduced distal nephron flow should be suspected.

Hyperkalemia is not always due to in vivo release of potassium and pseudohyperkalemia should be ruled out as first step in evaluation.

CAUSES OF HYPERKALEMIA

Pseudohyperkalemia (Fig. 8.1)

Pseudohyperkalemia represents an artificially elevated K^+ concentration in the plasma. This is due to K^+ movement from the cells immediately prior to or following venepuncture. When hyperkalemia is reported by the laboratory in an asymptomatic patient with no obvious underlying cause and no electrocardiographic abnormalities, pseudohyperkalemia should be considered.

Causes for in vitro increase of K^+ levels:

• Lysis of cells due to faulty blood collection procedures like excessive clenching of fist, prolonged tourniquet application during blood draw and Moisture in storage/ collection system.

Rupture of platelets

The normal serum potassium level is higher than the plasma K^+ due to K^+ release during clot formation. Platelets rupture due to clotting or contact with glass surface Rise in K^+ contributed by lysis of normal number of platelets is only 0.06 mmol/L.

There is increased chance of rupture if platelet size is large or platelet count exceeds normal range by more than $500,000/mm^3$).

- For every 100,000/mL increase in the platelet count, the serum K^+ increases by approximately 0.15 mEq/L. These phenomena can be seen normally in people who have leakier cell membranes.
- **Rupture of leukocytes** in conditions associated with WBC count more than 70,000/mm³ as in leukemias, circulating WBCs can be very fragile and rupture. This will release K^+.
- Erythrocytosis (hematocrit > 55%) can also rarely cause increase in K^+ levels.

To rule out Pseudohyperkalemia blood should be drawn into two tubes one by the usual technique and another sample from femoral vein or artery using a heparinized silicone-coated tube. Blood must be separated immediately to avoid in vitro release of K. In *Pseudohyperkalemia though serum K is high, plasma concentration of potassium will be normal.*

Case History 1

A 15-year-old child is admitted with fever and myalgia. Laboratory parameters are as follows:

Parameter in plasma/blood	
Total count	15000/cmm
Platelet count	500000/cmm
FBS	90 mg%
Urea	30 mg%
Creatinine	1.2 mg%
Na	140 mmol/L
K	5.5 mmol/L

Significant biochemical abnormality was a **serum potassium of 5.5 mmol/L.** Since, there was no obvious underlying cause and no electrocardiographic abnormalities pseudohyperkalemia should be considered.

In the above patient potassium estimation was repeated without a tourniquet and in heparinized sample. Serum K was 5 mmol/L, and this was pseudohyperkalemia

---

Causes of redistribution of potassium ICF to ECF are shown below (Fig. 8.2).

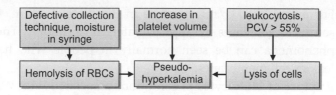

Fig. 8.1: Causes of pseudohyperkalemia

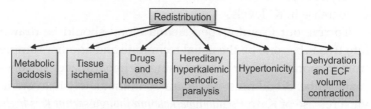

Fig. 8.2: Redistribution of potassium due to transcellular shift

The mechanism for secretion of K⁺ is intact till GFR falls to 25 mL/min. Potassium level will be brought back to normal by increasing the excretion of potassium even if shift of potassium occurs from ICF to ECF. But when GFR is less than 25 mL/minute, conditions that can cause redistribution can result in rise in ECF potassium.

CONDITIONS PRODUCING TRANSCELLULAR SHIFT AND REDISTRIBUTION OF K⁺ FROM ICF TO ECF

1. **Acidosis** Potassium gets redistributed in a variable fashion in various types of acidosis
   a. **Type of acidosis—respiratory or metabolic.**
      Metabolic acidosis is more commonly associated with high potassium.
   b. **Type of metabolic acidosis—**mineral acid (non-anion gap) or organic acid anions (high anion gap). Mechanism of hyperkalemia - In acidosis, H⁺ enters the cell, and the cell becomes more positive. To maintain

electroneutrality, either an anion has to accompany the H^+ ion or another intracellular cation K^+ has to leave the cell. Hyperkalemia is caused when the anion is not permeable to the cell.

In normal anion gap metabolic acidosis mineral acid anions like Cl^-, PO_4, SO_4^- accumulate. These ions are impermeable to cells and hence cannot accompany H^+. To maintain electroneutrality, K^+ leaves the cell resulting in hyperkalemia. A rough formula is **for every 0.1 change in** pH, serum potassium will change in **the opposite direction by 0.6 mmol/L.**

In anion gap metabolic acidosis, there is accumulation of organic acids like lactate, ketoacetate, etc. in the ECF. Organic anions enter the cells along with H^+ ions. This maintains the electroneutrality in the cell. So K^+ does not move from the cell to the ECF in exchange for H^+. One exception is diabetic ketoacidosis where anion gap acidosis can be associated with hyperkalemia. Cause of hyperkalemia is multifactorial and not due to acidosis alone. Hyperglycemia results in extracellular hypertonicity. When ECF becomes hypertonic, hyperkalemia is caused by 2 mechanisms:

i. Loss of intracellular water, resulting in an increased intracellular potassium concentration, favoring a gradient for potassium to move out of the cells

ii. As water exits the cells, —"solvent drag," sweeps potassium along. Other common causes of hypertonicity are hyperglycemia, hypernatremia and hypertonic mannitol. Hyperkalemia due to this is not severe unless there are confounding factors.

Duration of acidosis also influence the development of hyperkalemia.

2. Insulin deficiency or insulin resistance (i.e. type I or type II diabetes mellitus) results in impaired shift of K^+ from ECF to ICF.

3. Increased tissue breakdown—Internal hemorrhage and lysis of red cells in the body releases a large quantity of K^+ into the blood. In rhabdomyolysis, hypercatabolic states like sepsis, burns, etc. large scale tissue damage occurs and cell damage release K^+ from the intracellular compartment. Associated h potension, shock or sepsis may cause impaired K^+ excretion and aggravate hyperkalemia. Causes of *Rhabdomyolysis* are Heat stroke, chronic alcoholism, seizures, sudden excessive exertion (e.g. in military recruits undergoing rigorous training), or use of medications that interfere with heat dissipation (e.g. tricyclic antidepressants or anesthesia).

4. Tumor lysis syndrome—Ongoing treatment for widespread lymphoma, leukemia, or other large tumors can cause tumor lysis syndrome and release potassium from cells.

5. Massive hemolysis—Blood transfusion, sickle cell trait and hemolysis from any cause can release potassium from cells.

6. Drugs associated with transcellular shift
   a. Nonselective beta blockers (inhibits Na^+/K^+-ATPase pump).
   b. Digitalis (inhibits Na^+/K^+-ATPase pump).
   c. Succinylcholine (membrane leak).
   d. Sodium pump Inhibitors will impair K^+ entry into the cells and facilitate K^+ exit from the cells.
   e. Thalidomide in patients with preexisting renal insufficiency and as a complication in tumor lysis syndrome.

7. Aldosterone deficiency—Usual cause of hyperkalemia is diminished excretion of potassium in urine. Rarely long-term aldosterone deficiency impairs cell potassium uptake.

8. Hypertonicity—Hyperkalemia due to hypertonicity is caused by 2 mechanisms:

a. Loss of intracellular water, resulting in an increased intracellular potassium concentration, favoring a gradient for potassium to move out of the cells, and

b. As water exits the cells, "solvent drag," which sweeps potassium along. The common causes of hypertonicity are hyperglycemia, hypernatremia and hypertonic mannitol

Example: when one liter of water is lost from ICF volume of 30 liters, potassium will increase from 154 to 160 mmoles/L (by 1/30). There will be a parallel rise in serum potassium also.

9. **Hyperkalemic periodic paralysis** – Hyperkalemic periodic paralysis is a rare autosomal dominant disorder characterized by episodic weakness or paralysis, precipitated by stimuli that normally lead to hyperkalemia. (e.g., exercise). The genetic defect appears to be a single amino acid substitution due to a mutation in the gene for the skeletal muscle Na^+ channel.

10. **Dehydration and severe intravascular contraction** critically ill patients may develop hyperkalemia due to movement of water and K^+ from the ICF to ECF compartment and failure of extra cellular to intracellular movement.

11. **Toxins inhibiting the reuptake of potassium from the extracellular space** – Ingestion of toad venom (*Bufo bufo gargarizans*) is a common folk remedy for strengthening the heart in South Eastern Asian countries. Bufadienolides are cardiac glycosides present in toad venom, having a similar structure and biochemical activity to digitalis and cardenolides. They cause hyperkalemia by binding to the alpha subunit of Na^+ -K^+ - ATPase, thus, inhibiting the reuptake of potassium from the extracellular space. This compound is identified in some aphrodisiacs and Chinese medications (e.g. chan su).

Case History 2

A 61-year old man weighing 70 kg with history of long standing type 2 diabetes mellitus is on treatment with insulin. He is admitted with dyspnea. He is on treatment with Losartan for hypertension. On examination he is acidotic, and BP is 160/90 mm Hg. Laboratory parameters are as follows.

Blood/plasma	Day 1	Day 3
Sugar	106 mg%	100 mg%
Urea	85 mg%	54 mg%
Creatinine	2 mg%	1.9 mg%
GFR- calculated	33 mL/min	
Na	138 mmol/L	139 mmol/L
K	7 mmol/L	6.1 mmol/L
Cl	116 mmol/L	114 mmol/L
HCO$_3$	13.5 mmol/L	15.3 mmol/L
AG	12.50	14
Osmolality	296 mOs/kg	295
Urine osmolality	450	460

Patient has a urine volume of 1.5 liters and GFR of 33 mL/min. When GFR is more than 30 mL/min and when urine volume is more than one liter, potassium excretion is sufficient to prevent rise in potassium. Hence, in this patient, low GFR alone cannot explain hyperkalemia. Increased intake of high potassium diet or drugs that interfere with K secretion may be the cause. His diet chart was reviewed and he was not on high potassium diet, but was taking Losartan potassium which is an angiotensin receptor blocking agent (ARB).

In such patients, redistribution as a cause should be excluded.

Step 1: Assess ABG Status

ABG Values		
pH	7.306	7.3
pCO$_2$	27.8 mm Hg	35.4
PaO$_2$	67 mm Hg	135
HCO$_3$	13.5 mmol/L	15.3 mmol/L
O$_2$sat	90%	98%
AG	9	10

ABG showed normal anion gap hyperchloremic metabolic acidosis (HCMA).
In this patient, ARB and Acidosis were responsible for hyperkalemia by causing transcellular shift from ICF to ECF.
Management Losartan was stopped. Since, K was 7, measures to shift K into the cells and K binding agents were started.

HYPERKALEMIA DUE TO REDUCED EXCRETION OF POTASSIUM

Hyperkalemia may occur because of the inability of the kidneys to excrete K^+. Estimation of urinary K^+ helps to identify these causes. Under normal conditions, if Serum K^+ rises, renal tubules will secrete more K^+ and K^+ in urine will be high. This will normalize serum K^+. This compensation can occur only when renal K^+ handling is normal. *In Hyperkalemia, if urine K^+ is >100mmol/L, renal handling is considered to be normal.*

RENAL CAUSES OF DECREASED K⁺ EXCRETION (FIG. 8.3)

1. *Decrease in GFR*
   Hyperkalemia due to reduction in GFR occurs only when GFR drops below 25–30 mL/min. Severe hyperkalemia at this level of renal function is usually associated with either exogenous source of K, endogenous release of K or use of drugs.

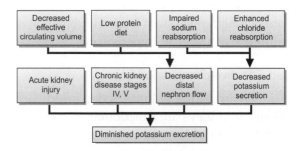

Fig. 8.3: Causes of decreased K secretion

2. *Decreased K secretion* — decreased distal nephron blood flow, impaired Na and Cl reabsorption, and endocrine causes can decrease K secretion and produce hyperkalemia. Most important and common cause of life-threatening hyperkalemia *is decreased urinary excretion of K.*

Acute Kidney Injury (AKI)

In acute kidney injury, inability of the kidneys to eliminate K^+ from the body results in hyperkalemia. The degree of hyperkalemia is more in older individuals, with concurrent use of drugs causing K^+ retention, inadvertent administration of K^+ in diet (fruits, tender coconut water), acidosis, shock or, severe dehydration. Careful attention to the diet and conservative treatment is sufficient in most cases. Hypercatabolism, transfusion especially of stored blood and packed red cell transfusions can contribute to sudden rise in potassium.

Hyperkalemia with AKI in such situations may require early dialytic support.

Chronic Kidney Disease (CKD) Stage IV/V

The ability of the kidney to maintain potassium homeostasis is preserved till the GFR is < 30 mL/min. Even in stage IV Patients who are on diet containing low K^+ and have urine volume more than 1 L potassium levels can be kept within normal range by conservative measures. This is due to the adaptive mechanisms in nephrons and GI tract. When GFR falls below 15–20 ml/min, hyperkalemia can occur even in the absence of a high potassium load. Combination of various factors culminate in a state of hyperkalemia.

Decreased Effective Circulating Volume

When effective circulating volume is decreased, GFR will be decreased and if kidneys are functioning normally, proximal tubular reabsorption of Na will be increased. This will result in reduced distal flow rate of sodium and water. K will not be secreted as no Na enters the cell. This can result in hyperkalemia.

Excessive dietary intake – Because the renal mechanism to excrete potassium is very efficient and K can be shifted to ICF, increased intake alone will not cause hyperkalemia. Hyperkalemia with increased intake is seen in patients with impaired renal excretion and or impaired intracellular shift.

Predisposing Factors

1. *High potassium, low sodium diets* – When protein is restricted in the diet, there will be increased intake of vegetables. Most of the vegetables are rich source of potassium and if not properly cooked, can release potassium and produce hyperkalemia in presence of low GFR.
2. Ingestion of potassium supplements.
3. High concentration of K in parenteral fluids.
4. Dietary salt substitutes – KCl instead of Na Cl.
5. Antibiotics containing K as penicillin potassium salt, amoxycillin clavulinate.

Case History 3

A 48-year-old man diagnosed to have diabetic nephropathy stage V was admitted with pleural effusion the day after hemodialysis. Investigations are as follows.

Parameters	Plasma
Sugar	200 mg%
Urea	180 mg%
Creatinine	12 mg%
GFR- calculated	4 mL/min
Na	141 mmol/L
K	6.3 mmol/L
Cl	103 mmol/L

Patient had hyperkalemia though he was on hemodialysis regularly.

What is the cause of hyperkalemia?

Is it due to transcellular shift? Drugs and other causes of transcellular shift were excluded.

ABG Values

pH	7.084
pCO_2	29.3 mm Hg
PaO_2	173 mm Hg on 40%O_2
HCO_3	8.5 mmol
O_2sat	90%

Diagnosis — Anion gap metabolic acidosis, (AGMA)
Respiratory acidosis
Hyperkalemia.
In AGMA, since H^+ ions enter the cell along with the organic anions, hyperkalemia is not as common as in HCMA. Hence acidosis alone is unlikely to be the cause for hyperkalemia.

The most common cause in such situation is intake of diet rich in K. Patient was hypercatabolic and diet records showed he had a high intake of K in the form of drumstick juice and tender coconut water. Probable cause is reduced removal of K in presence of increased intake. *Dietary counselling and intensive hemodialysis corrected hyperkalemia.*

Diminished Sercretion of K^+ as a Cause of Hyperkalemia May Occur with

1. Low aldosterone bioactivity due to adrenal insufficiency
2. Defect in secretion of K in CCD
3. Decreased effective circulating volume
4. Decreased urea (low protein diet).

Transtubular potassium gradient (TTKG) helps To differentiate between low aldosterone bioactivity due to adrenal insufficiency from defect in secretion of K^+ in CCD from other causes (Fig. 8.4).

TRANSTUBULAR POTASSIUM GRADIENT

The **transtubular potassium gradient** (**TTKG**) is an index reflecting the conservation of potassium in the cortical collecting ducts (CCD) of the kidneys. It is useful in diagnosing the

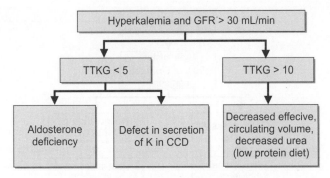

Fig. 8.4: Causes based on TTKG

causes of hyperkalemia or hypokalemia. The TTKG estimates the ratio of potassium in the lumen of the CCD to that in the peritubular capillaries.

The formula for calculating TTKG is shown below.

$$TTKG = \frac{Urinary\ K^+}{Urine\ osmolality} \times \frac{Plasma\ osmolality}{Plasma\ K^+}$$

TTKG is applicable only when the urinary osmolality is more than 300 mosmoles/kg.

The validity of this measurement falls on three assumptions:

1. Few solutes are reabsorbed in the medullary collecting duct (MCD).
2. Potassium is neither secreted nor reabsorbed in the MCD.
3. The osmolality of the fluid in the terminal CCD is known *(only in situations of profound K depletion or excess, significant reabsorption or secretion of K in the medullary collecting duct occurs)*.

TTKG in a normal person on a normal diet is 8–9.

When ECF K^+ increases due to whatever cause , to normalize plasma K^+, potassium excretion in urine will increase and the TTKG should be above 10. TTKG less than 5 in presence of hyperkalemia may indicate mineralocorticoid deficiency or defect in secretion of K at CCD.

Hyponatremia associated with increased Na excretion in urine may suggest mineralocorticoid deficiency.

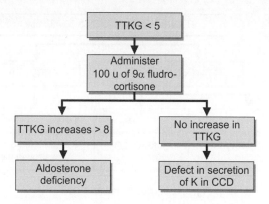

Fig. 8.5: Causes based on response to fludrocortisone

How to differentiate mineralocorticoid deficiency from defect in secretion of K at CCD?

If the low TTKG is because of low aldosterone bioactivity, physiological replacement dose of 100 µg of 9α Fludrocortisone should increase TTKG to >8. If TTKG does not show an increase after 9α Fludrocortisone, hyperkalemia is due to defect in secretion of K in CCD (Fig. 8.5).

ALDOSTERONE DEFICIENCY CAUSING HYPERKALEMIA

Aldosterone deficiency may occur in primary and secondary hypoaldosteronism or pseudohypoaldosteronism.

Primary Hypoaldosteronism

Causes

- Acute adrenal insufficiency (sepsis), or chronic adrenal insufficiency as in Addisons disease.
- Hereditary enzyme deficiencies leading to defective aldosterone biosynthesis.
  Defect in the enzymes 21 hydroxylase, aldosterone synthase, or 3 β OH steroid, dehydrogenase
  Clinical manifestations in children are failure to thrive, hyponatremia, hyperkalemia acidosis and hypertension.

Therapy with oral hydrocortisone and 9α fludrocortisone has been found to be beneficial.

Secondary Hypoaldosteronism

Renal Tubular Defects

1. *Type IV renal tubular acidosis:* Type IV RTA is more common than either type I or type II RTA. The most common cause of type IV RTA is hyporeninemic hypoaldosteronism.
   a. *The unique feature compared with other RTAs is hyperkalemia.* There is aldosterone deficiency or resistance. This will lead to impairment of cation exchange in the distal tubule with reduced secretion of both H^+ and K^+ and resultant hyperkalemia.
   b. Hyperkalemia induced impairment in ammonia production in the proximal tubule induces acidosis.
   c. Patients often have associated azotemia and hypertension. Because the distal tubule H^+ pump functions normally, in contrast to classical distal RTA, Urinary citrate may be normal or low.
   d. Associated renal dysfunction reduces secretion of calcium and uric acid, and stones do not form
   e. Therapy is typically directed at controlling the hyperkalemia.
2. *Hyporeninemic hypoaldosteronism:* Patients present with normal anion gap metabolic acidosis and hyperkalemia. The common causes are Diabetes mellitus, Tubulo-interstitial nephritis, Advanced age, systemic lupus erythematosus (SLE), Multiple myeloma and rarely acute glomerulonephritis.
   *Approximately 50% of patients present w*ith acidosis, reduced renal excretion of NH_4^+, and hence a positive urinary anion gap. Urine pH is < 5.5. When patients with CKD develop renal tubular acidosis, acidosis is out of proportion to the impairment in GFR.

3. *Aldosterone deficiency or tubular unresponsiveness to aldosterone:* There is impaired renal tubular potassium secretion and hence hyperkalemia.

Drugs Causing Hyperkalemia

Drugs cause hyperkalemia by many mechanisms β 2-adrenergic blockers, succinylcholine, digitalis overdose, hypertonic mannitol *cause redistribution of K⁺ to ICF compartment.*

Renin blockers, β blockers, Non- steroidal antiinflammatory drugs and cyclooxygenase 2 inhibitors,

Angiotensin converting enzyme inhibitors (ACE inhibitors).

Aldosterone antagonist, other K⁺ sparing diuretics

Aldosterone receptor blockers *act through renin angiotensin aldosterone axis.*

Angiotensin receptor blockers have less impact on circulating aldosterone level and so less chances of hyperkalemia.

Non-steroidal Anti-inflammatory Drugs and Cyclooxygenase 2 Inhibitors

Reduce renal blood flow and glomerular filtration rate. and they Inhibit prostaglandin causing indirect inhibition of renin release and aldosterone level. This effect is more in patients with pre-renal azotemia and congestive cardiac failure.

Heparin

Inhibits aldosterone synthesis. The unfractionated heparin cause more hyperkalemia than fractionated heparin.

Drugs Like Cyclosporin and Tacrolimus

Cause reduction in GFR and aldosterone secretion.

Aldosterone Antagonists (Spironolactone, Eplerenone)

Blocks aldosterone by binding competitively to mineralocorticoid receptors.

Case History 4

A 65-year-old gentleman with history of poorly controlled diabetes weighing 66 kg is admitted with obstructive nephropathy and urinary tract infection. On physical examination patient is euvolemic.
Laboratory parameters are as follows.

Parameters	Plasma
Sugar	152 mg%
Urea	46 mg%
Creatinine	1.3 mg%
eGFR/1.73 M^2	59 mL/min
Na	139 mmol/L
K	6.3 mmol/L
Cl	114 mmol/L
Albumin	3.5 g%
pH	7.38

What are the factors contributing to hyperkalemia?
Step 1: Exclude pseudohyperkalemia and excessive K$^+$ intake
This was excluded as there was no hemolysis, leukocytosis or thrombocytosis and blood was drawn without tourniquet and excessive clenching of fist. Patient does not give history of intake of diet rich in potassium. Hence, hyperkalemia is probably due to K shift from ICF to ECF and or decreased K excretion.
Step 2: *Assess ABG status This patient had normal pH*
As discussed earlier, patient should have some other factors to produce rise in K.
Step 3: To find out whether K excretion is adequate, estimate urinary potassium.

In presence of hyperkalemia, if tubules are responding normally, urine potassium should be more than 100 mol/L.

Urine Electrolytes

Sodium	77 mmol/L
Potassium	43 mmol/L

This patient had serum potassium of 6.3 mmol/L and 24 hr urine potassium was 43 mmol/L.

Step 4: Calculate TTKG:

$$TTKG = \frac{Urinary\ K^+}{Urine\ osmolality} \times \frac{Plasma\ osmolality}{Plasma\ K^+}$$

In this patient, plasma osmolality is 285 milliosmoles and urine osmolality is 394 mosmoles.

$$TTKG = \frac{43}{394} \times \frac{285}{6.3} = 4.9$$

TTKG < 5 indicated low aldosterone bioactivity or defective secretion of K+ in CCD

Patient was administered 100 μg of fludrocortisone and TTKG was repeated. TTKG was 6. Since TTKG is < 8, hyperkalemia was due to reduced secretion of K in CCD due to interstitial disease.

Failure of TTKG to increase after fludrocortisones can be seen with drugs (K⁺-sparing diuretics, trimethoprim, pentamidine), pseudohypoaldosteronism, Tubulo interstitial disease. *Potassium sparing diuretics (amiloride, triamterene)* block the apical Na^+ channel of the principal cell and their effects are independent of aldosterone. *Trimethoprim, pentamidine* impair K^+ secretion by blocking distal nephron Na^+ reabsorption.

Pseudohypoaldosteronism (PHA) Type 1

This is a condition characterized by normal blood pressure or hypotension, hyperkalemia, metabolic acidosis and have features suggestive of mineralocorticoid deficiency.

Forms of PHA **type 1**

1. Renal type I (renal PHA-I)
2. Multiple target organ defect type I (MTOD PHA-I)
3. Early childhood hyperkalemia.

Renal Pseudohypoaldosteronism Type I (PHA-1)

Renal PHA-I, or early childhood hyperkalemia, is probably due to a maturation disorder in the number or function of aldosterone receptors. This is an autosomal dominant disorder and has been associated with mutations in the human mineralocorticoid receptor gene (*MLR*). The renin and aldosterone levels are high and salt craving is more during stress. Salt supplements are continued till adult life and by adulthood, the extra salt requirement ceases.

Multiple Target Organ Defect Pseudohypoaldosteronism Type I (MTOD PHA-I)

Multiple target organ defect pseudohypoaldosteronism type I (MTOD PHA-I) is inherited as autosomal recessive trait. There is resistance to mineralocorticoid action in multiple body tissues. Other organs commonly involved are sweat glands, salivary glands and colon. The mutation of proteins controlling epithelial sodium channel ENaC results in defective Na transport in many organs containing the ENaC (e.g., kidney, lung, colon, sweat and salivary glands).

Degenerin/epithelial sodium channel (Deg/ENaC) super-family of ion channels is comprised of 3 homologous units (alpha, beta, gamma) and is expressed in the apical membrane of epithelial cells lining the airway, colon, and distal nephron. ENaC plays an essential role in transepithelial Na^+ and fluid balance. This is amiloride sensitive. The plasma aldosterone level is very high and such patients require strict potassium restriction and liberal sodium supplements. Since sepsis is common, antibiotic prophylaxis is advised. These children have high renin and aldosterone levels. This is due to ECF volume depletion and not due to aldosterone resistance.

Type 2 Pseudohypoaldosteronism (PHA)-II [Chloride Shunt (Gordon's) Syndrome]

PHA-II is a rare familial renal tubular defect inherited as autosomal dominant trait characterized by hypertension and hyperkalemic metabolic acidosis in the presence of low renin and aldosterone levels. The molecular basis for most individuals was linked to loss-of-function mutations in WNK1 or WNK4.

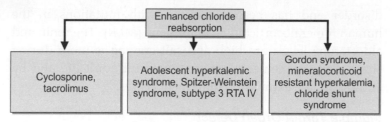

Fig. 8.6: Hyperkalemia with increased chloride reabsorption

WNKs comprise a family of serine-threonine protein kinases with unusual placement of the catalytic lysine compared with all other protein kinases. Two genes WNK1 and WNK4 are expressed in the convoluted tubules, collecting duct and the pumps in the segment.

Mutations of WNK4 increases the number of NCCT (thiazide sensitive sodium, chloride cotransporter), upregulates the renal outer medullary K^+ channel (ROMK) and epithelial channel. This results in sodium and K^+ retention leading to hypertension and hyperkalemia.

Mutation of WNK1 increases its expression and it suppresses WNK4 action. The plasma renin and aldosterone are reduced. Although hyperkalemia may be present from birth, hypertension develops in later life. Thiazide can be used to block the thiazide sensitive NCCT and reverse the abnormalities.

Adolescent hyperkalemic syndrome, Spitzer-Weinstein syndrome, subtype 3 RTA IV manifest in childhood and mode of inheritance is unknown. Other features are same as Gordon syndrome

Case History 5

A 3 month-old baby second child of non consanguineous marriage was admitted with incessant crying, vomiting, and skin rash. The baby is euvolemic and BP was 100/70 mm Hg. Laboratory parameters are shown below.

Blood/serum parameters	Values
RBS	90 mg%
Urea	15 mg%
Creatinine	0.6 mg%
Na	107 mmol /L
K	10 mmol/L
HCO_3	17 mmol/L
Chloride	80 mmol/L
Anion gap	10
Plasma osmolality	219 mOsm/kg

This child had severe hyponatremia, hyperkalemia.
What is the cause of hyperkalemia?
Is it due to reduce secretion of potassium?
Step 1: Measure urine electrolytes

Urine electrolytes in this patient

Urine sodium	52 mmol/L
Urine potassium	45 mmol/L
Urine osmolality	365 mOsm/kg

Urinary potassium is less than 100, indicating reduced secretion of potassium.
Step 2: Correlate with ABG

ABG values

pH	7.32
pCO_2	30 mm Hg
PaO_2	100 mm Hg on 21%O_2
HCO_3	15 mmol/L
O_{2sat}	90%

Patient has normal anion gap metabolic acidosis.
Step 3: Calculate TTKG
TTKG 45/(365 ÷ 219) ÷ 10 = 2.7

Low TTKG in presence of severe hyperkalemia was suggestive of low aldosterone bioactivity. Clinical and laboratory features were suggestive of pseudohypoaldosteronism. To differentiate type 1 from type 2 PHA, plasma renin and aldosterone levels were measured. Aldosterone was 1298 ng/L on normal sodium diet.

> Renin was 15.16 ng/mL/h. Diagnosis of PHA type 1 was confirmed. Child was treated with 20–25 g salt and sodium bicarbonate supplements. Hyperkalemia was managed with sodium polysterone sulphate retention enemas and the child improved.

TREATMENT OF HYPERKALEMIA

Acute rise in serum potassium is a medical emergency. Principles in the emergency management are:

Stabilization of Myocardium

If there is evidence of widening of QRS complex or other electrocardiographic evidence, antagonize the action of potassium on the myocardium by using calcium chloride/calcium gluconate slowly intravenously preferably under cardiac monitoring calcium stabilizes the myocardium from hyperkalemia induced arethmias.

Adult: Calcium chloride: 5 mL of 10% solution IV over 2 min or calcium gluconate: 10 mL of 10% solution IV over 2 min if available under cardiac monitoring (stop infusion if bradycardia develops).

Pediatric: Calcium chloride: 0.2 mL/kg/dose of 10% solution IV over 5 min; not to exceed 5 mL or calcium gluconate: 100 mg/kg (1 mL/kg) of 10% sol IV over 3–5 min; not to exceed 10 mL (stop infusion if bradycardia develops).

Calcium antagonizes cardiac, neurologic effects of hyperkalemia

- Second dose may be repeated after 5 minutes if there is no response
- Further calcium is ineffective unless hypocalcemia is also present
- Effect usually occurs within minutes and lasts for 30–60 minutes
- Anticipate EKG improvement within 3 minutes
- Use slower infusion (over 20–30 minutes)

- Caution in digoxin toxicity which may be worsened by hypokalemia
- Consider magnesium as alternative to calcium.

Shift of ECF Potassium to ICF

Potassium shift from intravascular to intracellular fluid

1. *Glucose and insulin infusion:* This will increase cellular K^+ uptake by stimulating the glucose−ATPase and thereby K^+ ATPase. Along with glucose, potassium also will shift into cells. Regular insulin 10 units IV, is given. If serum glucose < 250 mg/dL. 50% of 50 mL glucose is indicated with insulin. Give one ampule IV over 5 minutes. Consider maintenance (e.g., 5% dextrose, half normal saline 100 cc/h) post initial bolus to cover further insulin. Alternatively administration of 100 mL of 25% dextrose with 6 units of insulin can also be given as an infusion in 20 to 30 minutes. *Onset of action is within 15–30 minutes, and action lasts for 2–6 hours. Glucose is to be monitored frequently.*

   In pediatric age group, dose is 0.5 g/kg (2 mL/kg) 25% dextrose solution with 0.1 U/kg regular insulin (1 U regular insulin/5 g glucose) IV over 30 minutes.

2. *Beta 2-adrenergic agonists:* These agents promote cellular reuptake of potassium, possibly via the cyclic gAMP receptor cascade. Albuterol (ventolin, proventil, salbutamol) are adrenergic agonists that increases plasma insulin concentration, which may in turn help shift K^+ into intracellular space.

   This lowers K^+ level by 0.5–1.5 mEq/L and can be very beneficial in patients with renal failure when fluid overload is a concern.

   Adult dose is 5 mg mixed with 3 mL of isotonic saline via high-flow nebulizer every 20–30 minute as tolerated.

   In pediatric age group < 1 year: dose is 0.05–0.15 mg/kg/dose with 3 mL isotonic saline

   1–5 years: 1.25–2.5 mg/dose with 3 mL isotonic saline

5–12 years: 2.5 mg/dose with 3 mL isotonic saline >12 years: 2.5–5 mg/dose with 3 mL isotonic saline

Administer 10–20 mg over 10 minutes, onset of action is within 15–30 minutes and duration is for 2–3 hours

3. *Alkalinizing agents:* When there is acidosis, to maintain ECF pH within safe limits, H^+ will shift into cells. To achieve electroneutrality, K^+ will move to ECF. With correction of acidosis K^+ will shift back to ICF.

   1 ampoule of sodium bicarbonate 7.5% providing 44.6 meq is given IV over 5 minutes, or may be added to glucose infusion. It should never be used with calcium. The syringe and needle used for calcium should be replaced or flushed with sterile saline.

   Pediatric dose – Infants: 0.5 mEq/kg IV over 5–10 minutes; repeat in 10 minutes (**only use 4.2% solution,** not 8.4% solution usually used in older children and adults)

   Children: 1–2 mEq/kg IV over 5–10 minutes; repeat in 10 minutes

   a. Monitor ABGs - maintain arterial pH < 7.55

   b. May be repeated every 10–15 minutes if EKG changes persists

   c. Onset in 30 minutes

   d. Duration: 1–2 hours

   e. Avoid bicarbonate until hypocalcemia is corrected since there is risk of tetany and seizures.

Removal/Excretion of Excess of Total Body Potassium

This can be achieved by increasing the renal and fecal excretion of potassium

1. *Loop diuretics*: Frusemide given intravenously may be useful only if there is a diuretic response. The onset of action may be in 15–60 minutes, and duration is for 4 hours.

2. Cation exchange resins act by increasing K excretion through intestine. *Potassium binding resins* – Calcium polysterone sulphate is used.

Calcium polysterone sulphate is dissolved in water and then administered either orally (with the meal) or by retention enema. In the large intestine, potassium derived from food is exchanged for calcium ions. Finally, the indigestible potassium polystryene sulfonate complex is excreted with the feces, preventing the absorption of potassium into the blood stream. Hence, potassium is expelled from the body.

Recommended dose 15 g every six hours. In practice our patients respond to 5–10 g every six hours. This is dissolved in water, 4–5 mL per g of resin. In order to prevent constipation, this powder can also be dissolved in sorbitol. Sorbitol may be avoided in patients with risk for bowel necrosis.

Sodium polystyrene sulfonate (kayexalate) exchanges Na^+ for K^+ and binds it in gut, primarily in large intestine, decreasing total body potassium. Onset of action after oral administration ranges from 2–12 hours when administered rectally onset of action is longer. This lowers K^+ over 1–2 hours and duration of action is for 4–6 hours. Potassium level drops by approximately 0.5–1 mEq/L.

Pediatric dose: 1 g/kg/dose either orally or as rectal enemas are given. Multiple doses are usually necessary.

Dialysis

After instituting emergency measures for control of hyperkalemia, dialysis is useful in removing total body potassium. Hemodialysis achieves this by concentration gradient. Hemodialysis fluid contains only 2–2.5 mEq of potassium. In patients with hyperkalemia, potassium will move down the concentration gradient.

Peritoneal dialysis, solution contains 1.5 g% to 4.5 g% glucose depending on the type of fluid used. When glucose concentration increases in plasma, this will stimulate insulin and potassium will shift from ECF to ICF. Subsequently potassium moves down the concentration gradient into peritoneal cavity and results in lowering of total body potassium.

KEY POINTS

- Hyperkalemia greater than 6 mEq/L and or associated with ECG changes is a medical emergency and should be managed promptly.
- When there is no obvious cause, exclude pseudo-hyperkalemia.
- When GFR is more than 20 mL/min, high intake of dietary potassium, potassium containing medications, or potassium retaining drugs should be considered as the cause and should be withdrawn.
- Urinary potassium should be more than 100 mEq/day in presence of hyperkalemia and if less than 100 mEq, renal abnormality in excretion of potassium is the cause.
- TTKG will differentiate low aldosterone bioactivity from defect in secretion of potassium from low protein diet, low effective circulating volume.

Approach to hyperkalemia is summarized in Figure 8.7.

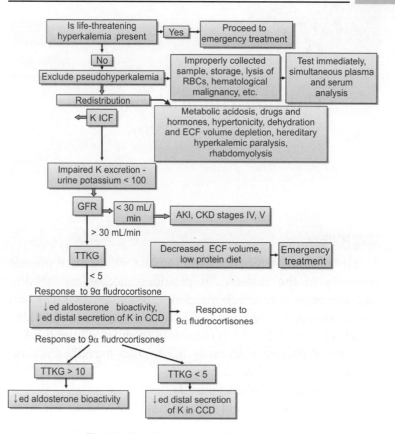

Fig. 8.7: Algorithmic approach to hyperkalemia

Calcium-Hypocalcemia and Hypercalcemia

A Vimala

OVERVIEW

Total body calcium (Ca) is around 1 to 2 kg. 99% of this is present normally in the skeleton. It provides mechanical stability and serves as a reservoir needed to maintain ECF calcium concentration. The remaining 0.5 to 1% is freely exchangeable with Ca in the ECF. 0.1% is present in the intracellular fluid.

Normal plasma calcium is 8.5 to 10.5 mg/dL. Calcium exists in plasma in three forms:

- Approximately 50% is ionized
- 40% is bound to mainly albumin and to a lesser extent to globulins
- 10% is loosely complexed with phosphate, sulfate, citrate and other anions.

Alterations in serum protein concentration directly affect the total plasma calcium concentration, but ionized calcium concentration remains normal. Corrected calcium can be calculated using the following formula:

Corrected serum Ca = [4 – patient's serum albumin] 0.8 + serum Ca

Change in pH can affect the concentration of ionized calcium. Acidosis also alters ionized calcium by reducing its binding with proteins. In alkalosis a large amount of calcium is bound to plasma proteins and ionized calcium is reduced. Patients with alkalosis are susceptible to hypocalcemic tetany.

Decrease in pH by 0.1 unit will increase ionized calcium approximately by 0.1 mg/L.

PHYSIOLOGY OF CALCIUM HANDLING

To maintain calcium balance, calcium intake should be equal to calcium excretion. Calcium is mainly excreted through GIT and kidneys. The physiologically important form of calcium is ionized calcium. When total plasma calcium increases there is increased binding of calcium to albumin and the ionized calcium is kept within normal limits. Similarly, when the albumin in plasma increase, the total calcium concentration decreases but the change in ionized calcium is minimal. The average Indian diet contains 1200 mg of calcium.

The reabsorption of calcium occurs mainly in the duodenum, jejunum, and ileum. In presence of oxalate or phosphate, calcium will combine with oxalate or phosphate and will become insoluble. This will be excreted in feces. Lactose will increase the absorption of calcium from the small intestine. Around 20 to 30% dietary calcium is absorbed. This is mainly regulated by 1,25, (OH), Vit D_3.

Parathormone (PTH) and Calcium Regulation

The most important regulator of calcium reabsorption is parathormone. PTH regulates plasma calcium concentration through three important mechanisms:
1. By stimulating bone reabsorption.
2. By stimulating activation of vitamin D, which then increases intestinal absorption of calcium.
3. By directly increasing renal tubular calcium reabsorption.

Renal Handling of Calcium

Calcium is filtered by the glomeruli and reabsorbed by the tubules.

Renal calcium excretion = filtered Ca – Ca reabsorbed.

Only about 50% of the plasma calcium exist in ionized form and is available for glomerular filtration. Normally, about 99%

of the filtered calcium is reabsorbed by the tubules, with only about 1% of the filtered being excreted. 65% of the filtered calcium is passively reabsorbed in the proximal tubulethrough paracellular route. This is linked to the reabsorption of Na and Chloride. This is not under hormonal control., 25 to 30% is reabsorbed in the ascending limb of loop of Henle by paracellular mechanism and 4 to 9% is reabsorbed in the distal and collecting tubules by transcellular mechanisms.

The lumen positive voltage drives calcium reabsorption and this is the main site of the regulation for urine calcium excretion. The reabsorption of the calcium is active in the segment.

Compensatory responses to decreased plasma ionized calcium concentration is mediated by PTH and vitamin D (Fig. 9.1). With an increase in calcium intake, there is also increased renal calcium excretion although much of the increase of calcium intake is eliminated in the feces. With calcium depletion, calcium excretion by the kidneys decreases as a result of enhanced tubular reabsorption.

One of the primary regulator of renal tubular calcium reabsorption is PTH (Fig. 9.1). With increased levels of PTH, there is increased calcium reabsorption in the thick ascending loop of henle and distal tubules, which reduces urinary excretion of calcium.

Reduction of PTH promotes calcium excretion by decreasing reabsorption in the loop of Henle and distal tubules.

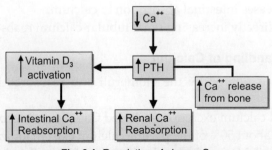

Fig. 9.1: Regulation of plasma Ca

Factors Decreasing Ca Reabsorption Leading to Increased Ca Excretion in Urine

1. Calcium reabsorption usually parallels sodium and water reabsorption. Factors which decrease Na^+ and H_2O reabsorption are extracellular volume expansion, increased arterial pressure will decrease calcium reabsorption from the proximal tubules.
2. Decrease in plasma phosphate suppresses PTH and reduce calcium reabsorption.
3. Metabolic alkalosis also will decrease calcium reabsorption.

Factors Increasing Ca Reabsorption Leading to Decreased Ca Excretion in Urine

1. Extracellular volume contraction or decreased blood pressure will stimulate increased proximal tubular reabsorption of Na^+ Cl^- and thereby increased calcium reabsorption.
2. An increase in plasma phosphate stimulates PTH, which increases calcium reabsorption by the renal tubules, thereby reducing calcium excretion.
3. Metabolic acidosis: Most of the effect of hydrogen ion on calcium excretion results from changes in calcium reabsorption in the distal tubule.

HYPOCALCEMIA

This is defined as serum calcium below 8.4 mg (normal calcium is 8.4–10.3 mg/dL).

When calcium ion concentration falls to low levels, the excitability of nerve and muscle cells increases markedly and in extreme cases results in hypocalcemic tetany. This is characterized by spastic skeletal muscle contraction.

Clinical features are:
- Chvostek's sign: facial twitch after a gentle tapping over the facial nerve (can occur in 10%–25% of normal adults)

- Trousseau's sign: carpopedal spasm after inflation of BP cuff above the patient's systolic BP for 2- to 3-minute duration
- Tetany, paresthesias, myopathy, seizures, muscle spasm or weakness
- Psychiatric disturbances: Psychosis, depression, impaired cognitive function
- Soft tissue calcifications, ocular cataracts
- Cardiac arrhythmias, congestive heart failure caused by decrease in myocardial contractility, increased QT interval and hypotension.

CAUSES OF HYPOCALCEMIA ARE EITHER DUE TO DECREASE IN PTH AND/OR VITAMIN D DEFICIENCY

1. Decrease in PTH

a. Hereditary hypoparathyroidism
b. Acquired hypoparathyroidism—post surgery
c. Hypomagnesemia—induces PTH deficiency
d. Renal disease usually with GFR < 30 mL/min
   i. Poor activity of renal 1 α hydroxylase
   ii. Decreased renal phosphate excretion
   iii. Excessive loss of 25 (OH) Vitamin D_3 in nephrotic syndrome

2. Causes for Vitamin D Deficiency

Lack of Vitamin D

a. Indequate dietary intake of vitamin D
b. Malabsorption of vitamin D
c. Lack of sun exposure:
   - Decreased hepatic synthesis of 25 (OH) vitamin D_3
   - Defective metabolism:
     Anticonvulsant therapy will increase cytochrome P-450 enzyme and increase hepatic catabolism of 25 (OH) Vitamin D_3.

Vitamin D Dependent Rickets

Type I and type II
- Pseudohypoparathyroidism: Peripheral end-organ resistance to PTH.

Risk of Hypocalcemia

1. Chronic hypocalcemia in patients with end-stage renal disease has increased risk for development of new and recurrent ischemic heart disease, cardiac failure. This is associated with excess mortality.
2. Vitamin D deficiency related hypocalcemia is associated with osteopenia and osteoporosis. Older women with vitamin D deficiency have a two fold increase in the risk of hip fracture.

Management of Hypocalcemia

Acute, symptomatic hypocalcemia is a medical emergency.
1. Treatment is initiated with 1 to 2 g of bolus dose of calcium gluconate given intravenously over 10 to 20 minutes followed by a slow infusion of calcium gluconate at 0.5 to 1.5 mg/kg/h.
   Calcium gluconate usually is preferred over calcium chloride because it is less likely to cause tissue necrosis if extravasated.
   Calcium gluconate intravenous preparation:
   I mL contains 100 mg
   Adults: 500 mg – 2 g (5–20 mL)
   Children: 200–500 mg (2–5 mL)
   Infants: 100 to 200 mg (1–2 mL).
2. Increase gastrointestinal absorption of calcium with calcitriol. Start at 0.25 µg twice a day and increase the dose after a couple of doses. Always replete the magnesium if low.

Chronic Hypocalcemia Associated with Hypoparathyroidism

1. Oral calcium: Calcium carbonate 1000 mg 3 to 4 times per day.
2. Calcitriol: 0.25 µg 3 times per day to maintain serum calcium in low normal range—8–8.5 mg/L.

Chronic hypocalcemia associated with vitamin D deficiency and hypophosphatemia should be treated with oral calcium supplementation and vitamin D.

1. Ergocalciferol (vitamin D_2) is given once weekly as 50,000 International Units orally or parenterally till replete. It is cheap but is metabolized by the liver and kidneys. It has a slow onset and long duration of action.
2. Calcidiol (25-hydroxy vitamin D) is available in capsules of 20 and 50 µg. Its action is more rapid and not as prolonged as that of ergocalciferol.
3. Calcitriol (1, 25-dihydroxy vitamin D_3) has the most rapid onset within hours and a shorter duration of action with half-life 4 to 6 hours. This does not require endogenous activation.

Chronic Hypocalcemia Associated with Renal Insufficiency and Hyperphosphatemia

- Vitamin D supplementation after reducing levels of phosphates.
- Oral phosphate binders (calcium carbonate, calcium acetate, sevelamer hydrochloride or carbonate, lanthanum) should be given to reduce phosphate levels.
- Calcitriol or another vitamin D analog.
- Cinacalcet is a calcimimetic agent for secondary hyperparathyroidism in patients with renal disorders. It has been shown to lower parathyroid hormone levels and improve calcium-phosphate homeostasis in comparison to placebo.

HYPERCALCEMIA

This is defined as serum calcium more than 10.3 mg/dL (normal calcium 8.4-10.3 mg/dL).

Causes of hypercalcemia can be due to increase in parathormone, excess of vitamin D, due to increased bone turn over or associated with renal failure.

Parathyroid Related

1. Primary hyperparathyroidism
   a. Solitary adenomas
   b. Multiple endocrine neoplasia
2. Lithium therapy
3. Familial hypocalciuric hypercalcemia.

Malignancy Related

1. Solid tumor with metastases (breast)
2. Solid tumor with humoral mediation of hypercalcemia (lung, kidney)
3. Hematologic malignancies (multiple myeloma, lymphoma, leukemia).

Vitamin D Related

1. Vitamin D intoxication
2. Increased 25 $(OH)_2$, Vitamin D_3, sarcoidosis and other granulomatous diseases.
3. Idiopathic hypercalcemia of infancy.

Associated with high bone turn over

1. Hyperthyroidism
2. Immobilization
3. Thiazides
4. Vitamin D intoxication.

Associated with renal failure

1. Teritiary hyperparathyroidism
2. Aluminum intoxication
3. Milk- alkali syndrome.

SYMPTOMS OF HYPERCALCEMIA

Patients are usually asymptomatic can present with non-specific symptoms like confusion, lethargy and obtundation, more common in elderly. Chronic hypercalcemia results in anxiety, memory disturbances and restlessness.

Patients can present with polyuria and this is due to loss of concentrating capacity of tubules. Polyuria can cause volume depletion. These changes stimulate proximal Ca reabsorption and worsen hypercalcemia.

Patients can present with nephrolithiasis as in hyperparathyroidism or sarcoidosis. Patients can present with acute kidney injury: The causes of acute kidney injury are decrease in GFR due to tubular damage from Ca deposition and also due to vasoconstrictive action. Urinalysis is normal.

Ultrasonogram may reveal nephrocalcinosis in chronic hypercalcemia and medullary sponge kidney.

- Patient can present with proximal myopathy
- Electrocardiogram (ECG) may show shortening of Q T interval and ventricular arrythmias.

MANAGEMENT OF HYPERCALCEMIA

Mainstay of management is volume expansion
1. ECF volume is expanded with saline infusion. This will reduce Na^+ and Cl^- reabsorption from proximal tubules. This will decrease passively the reabsorption of calcium. 4 to 5 L of normal saline can be infused over 24 hours. *Volume expansion is contraindicated in renal failure and congestive heart failure.*
2. Frusemide is given before administration of normal saline. This will block Ca reabsorption in the thick ascending limb. *It should only be used with volume expansion.* Administration of frusemide alone can cause ECF volume contraction and result in increase in proximal Ca reabsorption.
3. Calcitonin will decrease calcium by blocking osteoclast resorption.

4. Etidronate and bisphosphonate such as pamidronate–7.5 mg/kg/day intravenously over several hours daily for 3 days can reduce plasma calcium levels.
5. Phosphates can reduce calcium level by inhibiting the absorption of calcium from the gut by binding to calcium. This can also inhibit bone resorption.
6. Glucocorticiods are used when hypercalcemia is associated with hypervitaminosis A, D and sarcoidosis.
7. Hemodialysis is indicated in hypercalcemia when there is acute kidney injury.

KEY POINTS

- Physiologically active form of calcium is ionized calcium.
- Calcium is mainly regulated by parathormone and 1, 25-dihydroxy vitamin D_3.
- Extracellular fluid volume, blood pressure, plasma phosphate levels and arterial pH are important factors controlling calcium reabsorption.
- Acute symptomatic hypocalcemia is a medical emergency, and should be corrected with parenteral calcium gluconate.
- Hypercalcemia is also a medical emergency and should be treated with saline infusion and if required with other measures.

Section 2

Approach to Respiratory Acid-Base Disorders

- Overview and pulmonary physiology
- Analysis of respiratory acid-base status
- Therapeutic considerations in respiratory acid-base disorders
- Worked examples — Clinical problem solving

Overview and Pulmonary Physiology

G Krishnakumar

Acid-Base disorders of respiratory origin are due to primary abnormalities in gas exchange. These disturbances can result from disorders in ventilation, diffusion, perfusion or ventilation perfusion mismatch. Hypoxia and hypoxemia can be due to different causes and is briefly discussed below. In respiratory acid-base disorders theprimary change occurs in PCO_2 — an increase in PCO_2 in respiratory acidosis and a decrease in respiratory alkalosis. Metabolic derangements can also bring changes in PCO_2, hence an abnormal PCO_2 should be interpreted in conjunction with HCO_3. Normal factors controlling respiration are PCO_2, H^+ ions, and PO_2. Acute changes in gas exchange produce rapid changes in pH in contrast to metabolic disorders where it takes time to manifest. This is because when changes in PCO_2 occur, pH is brought back to normal by reabsorption and regeneration of bicarbonate and changes in excretion of NH_3 which takes time. For better understanding of the above changes, a very brief review of pulmonary physiology is given.

COMMON ABBREVIATIONS

Hb - hemoglobin
PAO_2 – partial pressure of oxygen in alveolar air
PaO_2 – partial pressure of oxygen in arterial blood
$PACO_2$ – partial pressure of carbon dioxide in alveolar air

$PaCO_2$ – partial pressure of carbon dioxide in arterial blood
$A\text{-}aDO_2$ – alveolar-arterial oxygen difference

The lungs play an important role in oxygenation and elimination of carbon dioxide. Respiratory control of acid-base balance is mainly by control of PCO_2 which is determined by alveolar ventilation.

LUNGS FUNCTIONS

The primary function of the lungs is the transfer of oxygen from inspired air into the blood and carbon dioxide in the opposite direction. For this, there is a very large area (50–100 m²) of interface, the pulmonary alveolar-capillary membrane, between air in the alveoli and blood in the surrounding capillaries, for diffusion of gases in either direction.

The air pump consisting of the chest wall, intercostal muscles and diaphragm moves the gases over the membrane. The right ventricle maintains the flow of blood on the opposite side of the membrane. The constant flow of blood and the continuous replenishment of alveolar air are essential for proper oxygenation and carbon dioxide removal.

The simplified diagram of the lung (Fig. 10.1) shown below gives approximate values for gas and blood flows.

The hypothetical lung has a tidal volume of 500 mL and a breathing rate of 15 breaths/min giving a minute ventilation of

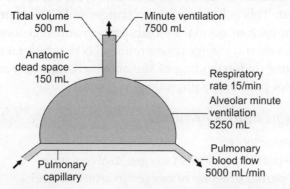

Fig. 10.1: Simplified lung unit (adapted from West 2000)

7.5 liters. 150 mL of air is unavailable for gas exchange (dead space) leaving us an alveolar minute ventilation of 5250 mL (350 × 17). Cardiac output (and therefore pulmonary blood flow) is 5 liters per minute. Note that the ratio of alveolar minute ventilation to pulmonary blood flow is close to 1:1, i.e. the ventilation perfusion ratio (V/Q) is one.

Ventilation

Tidal volume is the volume of air inhaled or exhaled in each breath. The volume of expired air in each breath normally equals the volume of inspired air.

Minute ventilation is the volume of air breathed in or out each minute (tidal volume (V_T) 500 mL × respiratory rate 15 breaths/min = 7500 mL in the figure above). The volume of air unavailable for gas exchange is *dead space* (V_D) 150 mL, so the part of V_T that is available for gas exchange is *alveolar ventilation*

$$V_A = V_T - V_D \text{ (500–150)} \times 15 = 5250 \text{ mL}$$

The only part of inhaled air that is involved in gas exchange is alveolar air. It is the part of total expired air that contains CO_2. Dead space not being involved, does not contain CO_2.

CO_2 being highly diffusible, its concentration in alveolar air is the same as in arterial blood ($PACO_2 = PaCO_2$, the small amount of CO_2 in inspired air being negligible). The amount of carbon dioxide produced must equal the amount of carbon dioxide that is excreted in expired alveolar air.

Since $PACO_2 = PaCO_2$, $PaCO_2$ must be determined by V_A. In other words *$PaCO_2$ varies inversely with alveolar minute ventilation.*

Total minute ventilation = tidal volume × respiratory rate

Anatomic dead space is the volume of the conducting airways where gas exchange does not occur.

Physiologic dead space is the volume of gas that does not eliminate CO_2.

Anatomic dead space = Physiologic dead space in normal subjects but physiologic dead space is increased in diseased lungs.

Physiology of Oxygen Transport in Blood (Fig. 10.2)

- Oxygen exists in blood as dissolved gas and in combination with hemoglobin.
- The quantity of oxygen that is dissolved in blood depends on its solubility in water and the partial pressure of the gas in alveolar air.
- The solubility of oxygen is 0.003 mL per mm Hg partial pressure per 100 ml blood, so normal arterial blood with a PO_2 of 100 mm Hg contains $0.003 \times 100 = 0.3$ mL of oxygen per 100 mL in the dissolved form.
- One gram of hemoglobin is capable of binding 1.34 mL of oxygen, so if a sample of arterial blood has 14g of Hb per 100 mL, it will be capable of carrying $1.34 \times 14 = 18.76$ mL of oxygen per 100 mL when fully saturated, i.e. carrying as much oxygen as it possibly can.
- Arterial blood is usually not fully saturated, so if it is say, 96% saturated it will carry $1.34 \times 14 \times 96/100 = 18.0096$ mL.
- The total *oxygen content* of blood in the above example is therefore
  (dissolved + oxyhemoglobin): $18.0096 + 0.3 = 18.3096$ mL/ 100 mL.

Oxygen saturation. Hemoglobin is fully saturated when all the available binding sites for all the hemoglobin molecules are occupied by molecule of O_2. Saturation is determined by

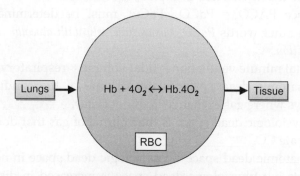

Fig. 10.2: Oxygen transport in blood

the partial pressure of oxygen but not in a linear fashion like solubility. The combination of each molecule of O_2 with the Hb molecule facilitates the attachment of an additional O_2, so that oxygen saturation (SO_2) is related to partial pressure of oxygen (PO_2) by a sigmoid curve (Fig. 10.3).

The affinity of hemoglobin for O_2 is affected by pH, carbon dioxide, temperature and red cell content of 2,3-diphosphoglycerate.

- *Bohr effect:* When H^+ ions are increased in plasma, they bind to Hb and decreases its affinity for O_2. During exercise there is increased production of lactic acid at tissue level. This helps to increase the delivery of O_2 to tissues.
- *Effect of CO_2*

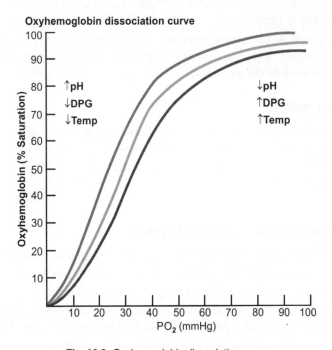

Fig. 10.3: Oxyhemoglobin dissociation curve

The CO_2 content of blood is higher in peripheral tissues than in pulmonary capillaries. This decreases the oxygen affinity of hemoglobin thereby helping to offload oxygen. When PCO_2 increases, there is increase in H^+ ions and CO_2 combines with amino group of globin to form carbamates (carbaminohemoglobin). These two mechanisms help release O_2 to tissues. Simultaneously, deoxygenation of blood in the peripheral tissues increases CO_2 uptake by blood *(Haldane effect)*. The PCO_2 difference between arterial and venous blood is small (~40 and 45 mm Hg) compared with the PO_2 arteriovenous difference (PaO_2 100 and P_vO_2 75 mm Hg).

- *Effect of 2, 3-DPG:* The affinity of Hb for O_2 is reduced because Hb has greater affinity for 2, 3-DPG. The signal for increase in 2, 3-DPG is alkalenemia. DPG binds to Hb in chronic hypoxia thereby helping unload O_2 to tissues.

- *Effect of Temperature*
  Rise in temperature decrease affinity of Hb to O_2. During vigorous exercise, locally temperature rises and O_2 is released to the muscles.

Oxygenation

Normal values of arterial oxygen tension are shown below

Neonates	50–75 mm Hg
Children, adults	75–100 mm Hg
Elderly	100–1/3rd of patient's age

Carbon Dioxide Transport in Blood

Carbon dioxide produced in the mitochondria by aerobic metabolism is carried by blood in the reverse direction to that of oxygen for elimination through the lungs. Unlike oxygen, it is highly soluble in water and readily combines with water to form carbonic acid (a process accelerated by carbonic anhydrase in red blood cells) which gets converted to bicarbonate:

$$CO_2 + H_2O \rightarrow H_2CO_3 \rightarrow H^+ + HCO_3^-$$

Carbon dioxide, therefore, exists in blood in 4 forms: as dissolved CO_2, carbonic acid, bicarbonate, and bound to hemoglobin as carbaminohemoglobin.

In arterial blood 90% of CO_2 is carried as bicarbonate and another major fraction as dissolved gas. Carbonic acid and carbaminohemoglobin account for only small fractions.

The above equation can be driven in both directions by changes in CO_2, H^+, or HCO_3 (buffering). Chemical buffering is instantaneous and can only affect the relative ratios of CO_2 and HCO_3, not their absolute quantities.

Large changes in total CO_2 content of blood can be made by the lungs over minutes by altering ventilation. The kidneys can decrease or increase reabsorption of HCO_3 more slowly and this takes two to three days. The CO_2 content of blood is higher in peripheral tissues than in pulmonary capillaries. This decreases the oxygen affinity of hemoglobin thereby helping to offload oxygen (Bohr effect).

Simultaneously, deoxygenation of blood in the peripheral tissues increases CO_2 uptake by blood (Haldane effect). The PCO_2 difference between arterial and venous blood is small (~40 and 45 mm Hg) compared with the PO_2 arteriovenous difference (PaO_2 100 and PvO_2 75 mm Hg).

CO_2 TRANSPORT (FIG. 10.4)

Ventilatory Control of Acid-Base

The body regulates its acid-base status through many mechanisms. There are various buffering systems at intracellular level, in interstitial fluid and in blood at the extracellular level.

Final adjustments are by the kidneys and the lungs. These adjustments are carried out regularly for variations in acid production as a result of metabolic changes and as compensations for changes due to disease processes.

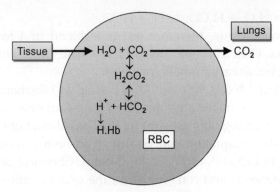

Fig. 10.4: CO_2 transport

The lungs work by regulation of carbon dioxide excretion. Large quantities of acid are produced in the body during normal metabolism — about 12,000–15,000 mmol per day of which only about 70–100 mmol is in the form of 'titrable acid' excretable by the kidneys. The remaining thousands of mmol of acid is in the form of carbon dioxide and is continuously excreted by the lungs. Thus, if the lungs were to stop working suddenly respiratory acidosis would ensue acutely in a matter of minutes while in acute renal failure acidosis takes about a day to manifest.

Carbon dioxide transport out of the body is directly proportional to alveolar minute ventilation (V_A) and CO_2 production is dependent on metabolic rate. Ventilation, therefore has to be closely matched to metabolic rate.

Control of Ventilation

In the normal human being, the control of ventilation is based on arterial PCO_2. V_A is so closely matched to CO_2 production that the $PaCO_2$ varies very little despite large variations in ventilation determined by rest and exercise. In exercise, CO_2 production is many times greater than during rest. If alveolar ventilation is to remain constant, a large increase in PCO_2 should occur during exercise. Since, alveolar ventilation increases with increased CO_2 production, PCO_2 remains within normal range. Such minute-by-minute control of respiratory activity is mediated by the central chemoreceptors situated in the floor of the 4th ventricle close to the medullary respiratory centre. The central chemoreceptors are responsive to changes · in [H^+] in the surrounding cerebrospinal fluid. Changes in CSF [H^+] occur rapidly in response to changes in arterial PCO_2 because CSF has very little buffering capacity compared to blood. The ventilatory response to $PaCO_2$ is normally rapid but may be blunted in sleep, old age, by drugs and disease states.

A decrease in arterial pH also causes an increase in ventilation independent of $PaCO_2$. An example is the Kussmaul breathing of diabetic ketoacidosis.

In patients with longstanding elevated arterial PCO_2 (chronic lung disease) the CSF pH is normal and changes little with change in ventilation. These patients are dependent on arterial PO_2 changes for control of respiration. The ventilatory response to hypoxia ('hypoxic drive') is not as sensitive as that to hypo/hypercarbia. In experiments in normal volunteers, the alveolar PO_2 could be reduced to 50 mm Hg before an increase in ventilation occurred ($PaCO_2$ being maintained at normal by adjusting the inhaled gas mixture).

As a consequence of the above:

H^+ and HCO_3 are produced 1:1 from CO_2, but ratio of concentration of H^+ to HCO_3 is 1: 10^6.

$PaCO_2$ will change with changes in CO_2 production in patients on fixed alveolar ventilation without patient trigger.

$PaCO_2$ will increase in patients being treated with Na HCO_3 for metabolic acidosis.

KEY POINTS

- The primary function of the lungs is transport of oxygen from air to blood and carbon dioxide in the opposite direction.
- Oxygen carriage in blood is largely due to its reversible attachment to hemoglobin. The affinity of hemoglobin for

O_2 varies with blood pH and PCO_2, so that it takes up more O_2 in the lungs and releases O_2 in peripheral tissues.

- $PaCO_2$ is inversely proportional to alveolar minute ventilation. Alveolar minute ventilation varies directly with CO_2 production.

- Carbon dioxide transport in blood is mostly in the form of bicarbonate.

Analysis of Respiratory Acid-Base Status

G Krishnakumar

Arterial blood gas measurement allows us to interpret the oxygenation status (PO_2) and the acid-base status (pH, PCO_2) of a patient. Interpretation of acid-base enables us to make deductions about the derangements in respiratory and metabolic function that may be present.

An acid-base nomogram indicating approximate reference values for common acid base disturbances is given in Figure 11.1. This is a graphical representation of the rules used to interpret clinical arterial blood gas values. The values can be inserted into the diagram and the diagnosis read directly.

OXYGENATION STATUS

The partial pressure of oxygen in arterial blood (PaO_2) is close to the partial pressure of oxygen in the pulmonary alveoli (PAO_2) in health. In disease processes affecting the respiratory system PAO_2 can be very different from PaO_2, i.e., the alveolar-arterial oxygen difference (A-a DO_2) may be increased. In most lung diseases, hypoxia can be corrected by administering oxygen. The severity of hypoxia in some lung diseases, particularly acute respiratory distress syndrome (ARDS, Table 11.1) means that often it is only partially corrected by administering oxygen, even if given by mechanical ventilator. Calculating the PaO_2/ FiO_2 ratio (the ratio of arterial oxygen tension to the fraction of oxygen in inspired air) enables assessment of severity of

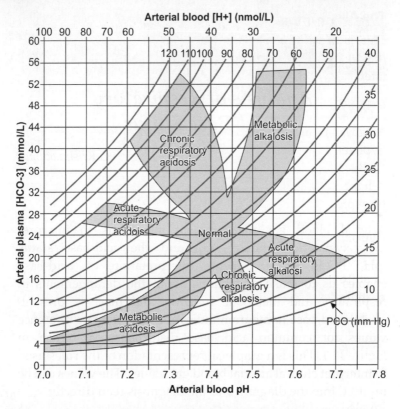

Fig. 11.1: Acid-Base nomogram

ARDS. A PaO_2/FiO_2 ratio of less than 300 mm Hg is a defining criterion for ARDS.

Table 11.1: Hypoxia in ARDS

PaO_2/FiO_2 ratio (mm Hg)	Comment
> 500	Normal
201–300	mild ARDS
101–200	moderate ARDS
<100	severe ARDS

The Alveolar-Arterial PO$_2$ Difference

This is the difference between alveolar ($P_{A}O_2$) and arterial (PaO_2) oxygen partial pressures. This is discussed in detail later.

HYPOXIA

Hypoxia — is defined as low O_2 tension in alveolar air, and hypoxemia is low O_2 in arterial blood.

By considering the idealised lung discussed earlier (Chapter 10), five possible mechanisms of arterial hypoxia can be explained:

Hypoxic Hypoxia

At sea level, atmospheric air contains 21% O_2. With increase in altitude O_2 tension decreases so inhaled air will have a low partial pressure of O_2. This 'hypoxic hypoxia' can be corrected by supplementing O_2.

Hypoventilation

Normal ventilation continuously replenishes alveolar air with O_2 and removes CO_2. When ventilation is not adequate, the inhaled air and thereby alveolar air cannot be replenished with O_2 and CO_2 cannot be removed. This can produce hypoxia. Hypoventilation invariably causes hypercarbia-increase in PCO_2 along with decrease in PaO_2. Hypoxia can be corrected with added inspired oxygen. But hypercarbia can be corrected only by increasing alveolar ventilation.

Diffusion Defect

As described earlier, alveolar-capillary membrane forms a large area of interface for gas exchange. In a diffusion defect, the membrane does not permit adequate gas exchange, with consequent hypoxia. Although theoretically possible, this is not of clinical importance.

Shunt

Normally, the venous blood from the tissues get oxygenated and enter the left side of the heart and aorta. In situations where there is mixing of venous and arterial blood, blood does not get oxygenated. This can occur within the lung or in the heart. Intracardiac shunts can cause hypoxia if high right heart pressures push venous blood into the left side of the heart and aorta-a situation that exists in cyanotic congenital heart disease. Hypoxia due to shunt does not get corrected by inhalation of 100% oxygen.

Ventilation-perfusion mismatch—air flow (V) and blood flow (Q) in alveoli in different parts of the lung do not match perfectly, some alveoli being under perfused and some perfused alveoli being underventilated. Even in the normal lung, the V/Q ratios are not the same in different parts, especially in the upright position. But the degree of mismatch is greater in disease states and this increased V/Q mismatch accounts for hypoxia and hypercarbia in a variety of lung diseases, most notably in the acute respiratory distress syndrome. Increasing overall ventilation (e.g. by intubation and mechanically assisting ventilation) often corrects the hypercarbia but only partially corrects the hypoxia.

Tissue Hypoxia

Decreased oxygen availability to the *tissues (tissue hypoxia)* can occur by the following mechanisms:
- Anemia reduces the oxygen carrying capacity of blood (carbon monoxide also does the same)
- Decreased cardiac output reduces the oxygen delivered to tissues
- Mitochondrial dysfunction or toxins such as cyanide impair oxygen utilisation.

A-aDO$_2$ (A – aO$_2$) can be used to find out the cause of hypoxemia

How is the A-aDO$_2$ Calculated?

This is the difference between alveolar (P$_A$O$_2$) and arterial (PaO$_2$) oxygen partial pressures. Since, it is not easy to sample alveolar air, P$_A$O$_2$ must be calculated. It depends on the partial pressure of oxygen in inspired air (PiO$_2$), the partial pressure of carbon dioxide in alveolar air, and the respiratory exchange ratio (also called the respiratory quotient, RQ).

PiO$_2$ in turn depends on barometric pressure, P$_B$, which at sea level is 760 mm Hg. When air passes through the nose, it gets fully saturated with water vapor and has 21% oxygen so PiO$_2$ = 21% of (760–47), 47 mm Hg being the saturation vapor pressure (SVP) of water. This gives us a PiO$_2$ of 149.7 mm Hg for a person breathing air at sea level.

In the alveolar air, the carbon dioxide that has diffused out from pulmonary capillary blood displaces some of the oxygen. P$_A$CO$_2$ is practically equal to PaCO$_2$ as CO$_2$ is highly diffusible. However the volume of CO$_2$ produced is less than the volume of O$_2$ inspired (the respiratory quotient, RQ) so this reduces the alveolar CO$_2$ volume by a factor equal to RQ.

The above considerations give us the alveolar gas equation:

$$P_AO_2 = FiO_2 (P_B - SVP) - PaCO_2/RQ$$

Worked out using typical values (150 mmHg for PiO$_2$ and 40 mmHg for PaCO$_2$), P$_A$O$_2$ = 150 – 40/0.8 = 100 mmHg

If the measured arterial PO$_2$ is 97 mmHg, the A – aO$_2$ difference is 3 mm Hg (100 – 97). Normal value is < 15.

Diagnostic Significance of A-aO$_2$

Respiratory failure can be due to neuromuscular diseases, chest wall abnormalities, diseases of pleura, airway obstruction etc. (hypoventilation causes hypoxia with hypercarbia) and intrinsic diseases of the lung (hypoxia and hypocarbia).

The A-a DO$_2$ enables us to understand how much of decrease in PaO$_2$ (hypoxemia) is contributed by changes in ventilation (low P$_A$O$_2$) and how much is due to defective transfer from the alveoli to blood (normal P$_A$O$_2$, low PaO$_2$).

With improvement in pulmonary condition, A-aO$_2$ will narrow.

Drawbacks

- The PO$_2$ of the inspired air should be known. In patient's breathing room air and on mechanical ventilators this is accurate. In patients on masks and nasal catheters, FiO$_2$ is not correctly known.
- A -aO$_2$ difference utilizes PO$_2$ and not O$_2$ content.
- Cardiac output has to be considered since this determines pulmonary AV shunt. This is not taken into consideration.
- A steady state is assumed.
- Respiratory quotient also will differ depending on the diet we eat.

Test your understanding: Calculate the alveolar-arterial PO$_2$ difference

1. FiO$_2$ 0.4, PaCO$_2$ 52 mm Hg, PaO$_2$ 160 mm Hg.
2. Breathless young man with PaCO$_2$ 20 mm Hg, PaO$_2$ 120 mm Hg on room air.
3. FiO$_2$ 0.8, PaCO$_2$ 38 mm Hg, PaO$_2$ 340 mm Hg in ventilated patient (assume patients are at sea level).

Answers

1. P$_A$O$_2$ = 0.4 (760 – 47) – (52/0.8) = (0.4 × 713) – 65 = 220
   A – aO$_2$ = 220 – 160 = 60 mm Hg. *Elevated alveolar-arterial O$_2$ tension difference, Hypoxia has been easily corrected with supplemented oxygen.*
2. P$_A$O$_2$ = P$_A$O$_2$ = 0.0.21 (760 – 47) – (200.8) = (0.21 × 713) – 25 = 125, PaO$_2$ – P$_a$O$_2$ = 5 mm Hg.
   Normal alveolar-arterial O$_2$ tension difference, Hypocapnia due to hyperventilation.
3. P$_A$O$_2$ = 0.8 (760 – 47) – (38/0.8) = (0.8 × 713) – 47.5 = 522.9
   PaO$_2$ = 523, PaO$_2$ – PaO$_2$ = 182 mm Hg. Indicates *Markedly abnormal oxygen exchange.*

Respiratory Acid-Base Disturbances

Various respiratory and metabolic disorders cause changes in hydrogen ion concentration, [H$^+$]. [H$^+$] is commonly expressed as pH, which is the negative logarithm of [H$^+$]. [H$^+$] in body fluids is extremely low, measurable in nanomoles per liter. Respiratory disorders change pH by causing primary changes in PCO$_2$.

$$H^+ + HCO_3 \leftrightarrow H_2O + CO_2$$

If there is an imbalance between production and elimination of CO$_2$, the resultant change in PaCO$_2$ will change the equilibrium in the equation.

Accumulation of CO$_2$ will increase H$^+$ ions and respiratory acidosis will ensue. The reverse happens when CO$_2$ decreases and respiratory alkalosis will result.

RESPIRATORY ACIDOSIS

As mentioned above, respiratory acidosis occurs as a result of CO$_2$ accumulation, i.e. hypoventilation inappropriate for CO$_2$ production. This can be due to:

- Central—respiratory depression, e.g. opioid effect, brainstem dysfunction.
- Neuromuscular dysfunction, e.g. myasthenia, Guillain-Barré syndrome.
- Decreased respiratory system compliance, e.g. stiff lungs in acute respiratory distress syndrome.
- Increased airway resistance, e.g. chronic obstructive airway disease.
- Controlled ventilation when alveolar minute ventilation is set at an inappropriately low value and the patient is too obtunded or sedated and/or paralyzed to trigger breaths.

Because renal compensation is slow, it is possible to differentiate acute from chronic respiratory acidosis (Figs. 11.2 to 11.4) by interpreting at the blood gas values according to the rules given in Table 11.2.

Unlike metabolic disorders, respiratory acidosis does not affect ECF electrolytes greatly. However, acidosis decreases

Table 11.2: Expected changes in bicarbonate and pH for a primary change in arterial carbon dioxide tension in respiratory acidosis

Change (for primary Δ PCO₂)	Acute respiratory acidosis	Chronic respiratory acidosis
Rise in HCO₃	1 mmol/L for each 10 mm Hg rise in PCO₂	3.5 to 4 mmol/L for each 10 mm Hg rise in PCO₂
Fall in pH	$0.008 \times (PaCO_2 - 40)$	$0.003 \times (PaCO_2 - 40)$

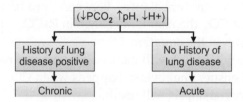

Fig. 11.2: Approach to respiratory acidosis

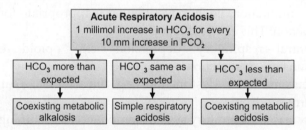

Fig. 11.3: Acute respiratory acidosis

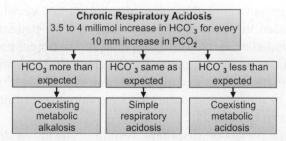

Fig. 11.4: Chronic respiratory acidosis

binding of calcium to albumin and tends to increase serum ionized calcium levels. It also tends to cause an extracellular shift of potassium, but respiratory acidosis rarely causes clinically significant hyperkalemia.

Clinically, respiratory acidosis can present with headache, restlessness, hypertension, tachycardia with a bounding pulse and warm extremities. If severe the neurologic symptoms can progress to generalized hyperreflexia, asterixis and coma (carbon dioxide narcosis). Papilledema can occur.

Treatment of respiratory acidosis is treatment of the underlying disorder. In ventilated patients, appropriate change in ventilator settings may be needed to correct hypoventilation.

Case History 1

A 75-year-old man with a long standing history of heavy smoking is brought to the hospital in a febrile and confused state. He rapidly becomes drowsy. SpO_2 is 80%.

Investigations

Na 134	K 5.0	Cl	82 mmol/L	HCO_3 29
ABGs	pH 7.21	PCO_2	70	PO_2 55

Clinical assessment indicates the patient is likely to have a chronic respiratory acidosis. He is hypoxic, so there is a possibility of lactic acidosis in addition.

ABGs: Patient is acidaemic, The change in pH is shifted in opposite direction to changes in PCO_2 and HCO_3 suggesting primary respiratory acidosis. Interpreting the values using the rules in Table 11.2 as follows:

The renal compensation for a chronic rise in PCO_2 of 30 (70 – 40) should be 3.5 × 3 = 10.5, so the HCO_3 should have been 24 + 10.5 = 34.5 mmol/L. There is therefore a metabolic acidosis also.

Anion gap is (134 + 5) – (82 + 29) = 28

The Δ ratio need not be calculated (we already know there is respiratory acidosis) and the bicarbonate is increased above the normal of 24, not decreased.

The patient has chronic respiratory acidosis due to chronic obstructive lung disease and metabolic acidosis due to possible lactic acid accumulation in hypoxia.

RESPIRATORY ALKALOSIS

Respiratory alkalosis results from hyperventilation—an increase in rate and/or depth of ventilation. This can result from:

- Hypoxia, e.g. high altitude, asthma, pulmonary embolism
- Central nervous system stimulation, e.g. stimulant drugs, anxiety, central neurogenic hyperventilation
- Miscellaneous, e.g. sepsis, recovery from metabolic acidosis. As with respiratory acidosis, acute and chronic respiratory alkalosis (Figs 11.5 to 11.7) can be distinguished by the extent of renal compensation (Table 11.3):

Acute respiratory alkalosis causes cerebral vasoconstriction that may cause lightheadedness and loss of consciousness. Perioral paraesthesia, syncope, cramps, carpopedal spasm and seizures can ensue from the fall in ionized calcium induced by alkalosis. Tachypnea or hyperpnea may be seen. Chronic respiratory alkalosis is usually asymptomatic.

Alkalosis causes a fall in ionized calcium because it increases the number of negatively charged binding sites on plasma proteins. Serum magnesium, phosphorus and potassium also fall because of intracellular shift of these ions. Respiratory alkalosis can be due to a primary condition causing hypoxia such as pulmonary embolism—which causes a raised alveolar-arterial O_2 gradient.

Treatment is treatment of the underlying cause. Respiratory alkalosis is not life-threatening, so interventions are not

Table 11.3: Expected change in bicarbonate and pH for primary change in carbon dioxide in respiratory alkalosis

Change (for primary Δ PCO₂)	Acute respiratory alkalosis	Chronic respiratory alkalosis
Fall in HCO₃ (max compensation 12–20 mmol/L)	2 mmol/L for each 10 mm Hg fall in PCO_2	4 mmol/L for each 10 mm Hg fall in PCO_2
Rise in pH	$0.008 \times (4\,0-PCO_2)$	$0.017 \times (4\,0-PCO_2)$

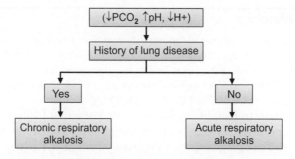

Fig. 11.5: Approach to respiratory alkalosis

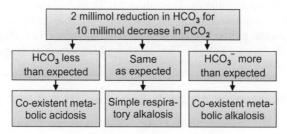

Fig. 11.6: Acute respiratory alkalosis

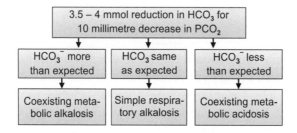

Fig. 11.7: Approach to chronic respiratory alkalosis
(Expected increase in pH is 0.003 U for every millimeter decrease in PCO_2)

required to lower pH. Increasing inspired CO_2 through rebreathing (such as from a paper bag) may be tried with caution.

Case History 2

A 28-year-old primigravida in her 7th month of pregnancy presents to Casualty with breathlessness and wheeze. She has had asthma in the past but no attacks since becoming pregnant. Her respiratory rate is 32/min and SPO_2 is 99%. Her arterial blood gas values:

  pH 7.48 PCO_2 30 PO_2 95 HCO_3 22

According to clinical assessment, this patient is likely to have respiratory alkalosis due to hyperventilation, secondary to her asthma and her pregnant state. Pregnancy being a hypercoagulable state a pulmonary embolism is possible but is unlikely since she is not hypoxic. Interpreting the ABGs using the rules in Table 11.3, both PCO_2 and HCO_3 are shifted in the same direction making a mixed disorder unlikely. The fall in HCO_3 is 2 (24 – 22) which is close to the expected change for the 8 mm Hg change in PCO_2.

The rise in pH corresponds to the PCO_2 ($0.008 \times 10 = 0.08$). The ABG values confirm the clinical diagnosis of acute respiratory alkalosis.

Acute Respiratory Alkalosis Based on pH and PCO_2

Example: In a patient with PCO_2 : 20 mm of Hg. Expected Δ in pH is $20 \times 0.008 = 0.16$. So the pH should be $7.4 + 0.16 = 7.56$.

Actual pH on ABG is 7.6 and suggest coexistent metabolic alkalosis.

KEY POINTS

- Hypoxia can be caused by a variety of mechanisms, the most important being hypoventilation and ventilation-perfusion mismatch. Calculating the alveolar-arterial oxygen difference helps to distinguish between hypoventilation and lung disease as causes for hypoxia.
- Respiratory acid-base disturbances are caused by changes in $PaCO_2$.
- Acute and chronic respiratory acid-base disorders can be distinguished because renal compensation for a respiratory disorder takes a few days.

Therapeutic Considerations in Respiratory Acid-Base Disorders

G Krishnakumar

Hypocapnia results from hyperventilation. CO_2 being the major driver of ventilation, a low $PaCO_2$ decreases ventilatory response. Hypocapnia occurs in normal people at high altitude, in metabolic acidosis as respiratory compensation, and neurogenic hyperventilation.

RESPIRATORY FAILURE

Respiratory failure may be defined in physiologic terms as a failure to maintain normal arterial blood gas tensions (PCO_2 = 38.3 ± 7.5 mm Hg, PO_2 being more difficult to define as it decreases with age). Clinically, respiratory failure is hypoxemia (arterial PO_2 < 55 mm Hg) or inadequate ventilation causing hypercapnia (arterial PCO_2 > 55 mm Hg) or both.

Hypoxemic respiratory failure occurs primarily in conditions affecting the lungs.

- Cardiogenic pulmonary edema
- Asthma and chronic obstructive lung disease
- Parenchymal lung diseases such as pneumonia, interstitial lung disease, lung hemorrhage
- Pulmonary vascular disease such as thromboembolism, air, fat or amniotic fluid emboli
- Acute respiratory distress syndrome—primary due to lung disease or secondary to sepsis, burns, pancreatitis, multiorgan dysfunction syndrome.

In the above conditions PaO_2 is decreased but $PaCO_2$ is not elevated but may be low, at least in the initial stages of the illness, indicating increased alveolar ventilation due to hypoxia.

Hypercapnic respiratory failure is generally a result of hypoventilation as can occur in

- Neuromuscular disorders such as myasthenia gravis, Guillain-Barré syndrome, poisoning, coma
- Chest wall disorders such as contusion, pneumothorax, pleural effusion, rib fracture, flail chest, abdominal distension.

Hypoventilation causes hypercapnia but hypoxia can occur as the disease progresses and is aggravated by the low alveolar O_2 tension (PaO_2) caused by the high $PaCO_2$.

Assisting Ventilation

Respiratory failure is treated by treating the underlying cause of the disorder, e.g. antibiotics for pneumonia and if needed to sustain life, artificial ventilation. Artificial mechanical ventilation may be needed if arterial hypoxia and/or hypercapnia occurs. The following discussion is not meant to be a guide to mechanical ventilation: It is only an outline of a complex subject.

Hypoxia (hypoxemia to be more precise, in order to distinguish true arterial hypoxia from that due to low inhaled O_2 tension) can be treated by

1. Increasing the concentration of oxygen in inhaled air.
2. Opening up collapsed alveoli (a process termed recruitment) by increasing the pressure at which O_2-air mixture is delivered to the airways—positive inspiratory pressure.
3. Keeping alveoli open—positive expiratory pressure (CPAP or PEEP).

2 and 3 increase mean alveolar pressure and also increase alveolar minute ventilation artificially.

In mechanically ventilated patients, hypoxia can be treated by all 3 measures.

Hypercapnia or hypocapnia can be treated by increasing or decreasing ventilation, i.e. by altering tidal volume or respiratory rate (since minute ventilation = tidal volume × rate).

MODES OF ASSISTED VENTILATION

(A brief overview of some different ventilatory modes. Not at all comprehensive)

Positive pressure ventilation (higher than atmospheric pressure) is almost invariably used in modern intensive care.

Non-invasive Ventilation (NIV) is used to assist breathing when the patient has a good respiratory effort, is conscious and able to maintain the airway. Two modes of NIV are used:

- Continuous positive airway pressure (CPAP) provides the same positive pressure during both inspiration and expiration. It can be provided with simple equipment needing only a high pressure source of oxygen and air.
- Bilevel positive airway pressure (BIPAP) is administered using a ventilator with circuitry to detect the patient's inspiratory and expiratory efforts and then to shift from a higher inspiratory to a lower expiratory pressure and vice versa. The machine performs this cycling in synchrony with the patients respiratory effort.

CPAP is ideal for hypoxia without hypercapnia — such as cardiogenic pulmonary edema and pneumonia while BIPAP is useful for patients with hypercapnia such as COPD where it assists in normalising PCO_2 by increasing tidal volume. CPAP is also useful for reopening atelectatic parts of lung in mucus plugging or diaphragmatic splinting due to abdominal surgery. The differences between these modes are indicated in the Figures 12.1 to 12.3.

NIV has some advantages in the initial management of respiratory failure:

- It does not require tracheal intubation and therefore avoids the need for sedation

- It may be cheaper and shorten hospital stay
- Permits intermittent discontinuation for feeding and oral toilet.

Disadvantages Include

- There is often a large leak of air between the patients face and the mask, requiring constant nursing to maintain the mask in position
- No protection against aspiration
- Limited tolerance of airway pressure.

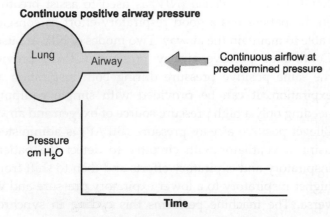

Fig. 12.1: Continuous positive airway pressure

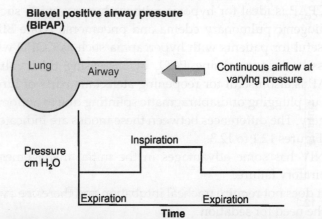

Fig. 12.2: Noninvasive ventilation with bilevel positive airway pressure

Invasive ventilation: This requires the use of sedation and endotracheal intubation for full airway control. This could become necessary, if the patient is mentally obtunded, is not maintaining adequate oxygenation on NIV, has severe lung disease such as acute respiratory distress syndrome, or other organ failures leading to respiratory failure. *Mechanical ventilators* deliver a flow of air through the endotracheal tube and the parameters for breathing can be set by the user:

- The pressure at which the lungs are inflated (inspiratory pressure, peak inspiratory pressure) in pressure control and pressure support modes (Fig. 12.3).
- The volume delivered (tidal volume and minute volume) in volume control/assist control and mandatory breaths in SIMV.
- The time during which inspiration occurs and expiration is allowed by the machine.
- A pause time between inspiration and expiration.
- Expiratory pressure (PEEP).

Expiration is passive, depending on the elastic recoil of the lungs and the ease with which the airways conduct alveolar gas to the outside. The machine has electronic control systems to sense the patient's effort and use this to begin and end each breath ('triggering') (Fig. 12.4). The machine can use this 'assist' mode in response to patient effort or can operate in a full 'control' mode where inspiration, expiration and cycling

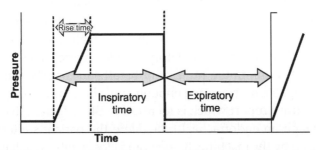

Fig. 12.3: Pressure—Time curve from a ventilator display showing inspiratory and expiratory times in pressure control mode

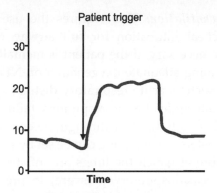

Fig. 12.4: Pressure-time curve showing dip in baseline pressure indicating patient triggered breath

between inspiration and expiration are all independent of patient effort and are set by the operator.

Different *modes* of ventilation exist, some of the common modes are:

• Volume control (assist control) where inspiratory (tidal) volume is set. The pressure required to achieve delivery of the set volume is dependent on the compliance of the lungs and resistance of the conducting airways. In this mode the pressures developed may be unacceptably high if the set volume is too high (see Fig. 12.5).

• Pressure control where inspiratory pressure is predetermined and the inspired volume depends on lung compliance.

• Mandatory modes where intermittent mandatory breaths at a set rate are administered in addition to patient actuated breaths. These mandatory breaths are usually synchronized to patient effort. Mandatory modes were devised to provide a minimum number of breaths in case the patient is incapable of triggering enough assist breaths on his own.

• Pressure support which is identical to BIPAP but delivered through an endotracheal tube. Here the patient's effort is sensed by the machine. It opens and closes valves to deliver a higher inspiratory pressure (IPAP) and a lower expiratory

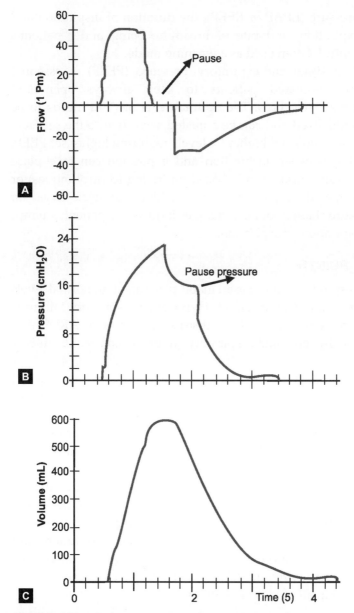

Fig. 12.5: A, Flow. **B,** pressure and **C,** volume-time curves from a ventilator in volume control mode. The flow is constant (flat-topped part of the flow-time and volume-time curves), inspiratory: Expiratory time is about 1:2 to allow for complete exhalation and there is no PEEP (pressure-time curve touches zero at end-expiration).

pressure (EPAP or PEEP), the duration of inspiration and expiration, and rate of breathing being under patient's control. Often used as a weaning mode.

A positive end-expiratory pressure (PEEP) is essential in all ventilated patients to keep airways open and minimize atelectasis. The optimal level of PEEP needs to be individualized and can be adjusted according to the set FiO_2, patients who need higher O_2 levels requiring higher set PEEP. Cycling between inspiration and expiration can take place either fully mechanically based on timing (control modes) or be triggered by patient effort: Machines can cycle based on pressure changes or flow changes induced by patient, attempt at inspiration or expiration.

KEY POINTS

- Respiratory failure is an inability to maintain normal levels of O_2 and CO_2 in blood. Hypoxemic respiratory failure is commonly due to lung disease (pneumonia, ARDS etc.) and hypercapnic respiratory failure is commonly due to hypoventilation.

- Respiratory failure can be treated by increasing inspired O_2 in hypoxic states and/or assisting ventilation in hypercapnia with hypoxia.

- Mechanical ventilatory assistance can be by means of non-invasive ventilation or invasive ventilation through an endotracheal tube. If the clinical situation permits, non-invasive ventilation is preferable to full invasive ventilation.

- Different modes of ventilation exist, differing in the extent of artificial control of breathing—inspiration pressure and volume, duration of inspiration and expiration, and patient initiation and termination of breaths. Positive end-expiratory pressure (PEEP) helps keep airways and alveoli open in all modes of ventilation.

Worked Examples—Clinical Problem Solving

A Vimala, G Krishnakumar

Case History 1

A 75-year-old 60 kg lady underwent hip surgery following a fall. She had been previously fit with no chronic illnesses and had been on no medication prior to the fall. She developed acute onset of dyspnea on the 3rd postoperative day.

What Could be the Cause of Her Dyspnea?

Differential Diagnosis

1. Lower limb large joint surgery is notorious for causing deep vein thrombosis (DVT) and subsequent pulmonary embolism, the highest incidence being reported with knee replacement. However, most patients now routinely receive prophylactic heparin.
2. Postoperative lung atelectasis is also quite a common complication in the elderly but is commoner with upper abdominal surgery.
3. A myocardial infarction or acute coronary syndrome can occur perioperatively when it carries a worse prognosis than in other settings.

   ECG showed an $S_1Q_3T_3$ pattern which taken together with echocardiogram that showed a mildly dilated right ventricle was considered to strongly suggest a diagnosis of acute pulmonary embolism.

How can a diagnosis of pulmonary embolism be confirmed?

The most useful test is a helical CT scan of the pulmonary arteries with CT angiography. Additional tests include:

- Doppler ultrasound of leg veins to demonstrate DVT
- D-dimer level for evidence of a clot (not useful in the postoperative patient)
- Radionuclide ventilation-perfusion scan.

She was given oxygen by mask but remained tachycardic, tachypneic and hypoxic (SPO_2 82%) in spite of increasing the oxygen concentration to 60% and was transferred to ICU for assisted ventilation.

ABGs on arrival:

pH 7.47 PCO_2 35 mm Hg PO_2 47 mm Hg HCO_3 26 mmol/L

Interpret These Values

Step 1: pH 7.47 is higher than the upper limit of normal pH 7.45, hence alkalosis.

Step 2: PCO_2 35 mm Hg is lower than lower limit of normal 40 mm Hg, hence respiratory alkalosis.

Step 3: History is suggestive of acute respiratory alkalosis. Expected HCO_3 is 23 (2 meq decrease for 10 mm Hg decrease in PCO_2), obtained HCO_3 is 26 meq/L, more than expected value – coexistant metabolic alkalosis.

Step 4: Find out the expected increase in pH 0.008 × decrease in PCO_2, 5 × 0.008 = 0. 04. 7.4 + 0.04 = 7.44, Here pH is more than expected also suggests coexistant metabolic alkalosis

Step 5: Interpret PaO_2 always in relation to FiO_2, patient on room air - FiO_2 0.21, PaO_2/FiO_2 = 47/0.21 = 235, suggests impaired gas exchange.

Step 6: Find out A- aO_2 difference

PAO_2 = (760 – 47) × 0.6 – (35/0.8) – 44 = 379, A – aO_2 = 379 – 47 = 332 mm Hg. The patient is hypoxic despite the high inspired oxygen and has $A-aDO_2$ more than 300 mm Hg, and in need of ventilator support. She is in respiratory alkalosis (high pH, low PCO_2) but the slightly elevated bicarbonate suggests the disorder is acute (lack of renal compensation) which we know to be the case and possibly also has coexistent metabolic alkalosis.

The patient was initiated on mechanical ventilation with a gratifying rise in the oxygen saturation. She was also started on IV heparin. Thrombolysis for the PE was not considered because of possible bleeding from the operative site.

The next morning the patient is mildly sedated, tachypneic (32 breaths/min) and on pressure support ventilation (PS 18 cm H_2O, PEEP 8 cm H_2O, VT 400 mL, FiO_2 0.6).

ABGs:

pH 7.26 PCO_2 65 mm Hg PO_2 60 mm Hg HCO_3 22 mmol/L

What is your Interpretation of the Above?

Step 1: pH 7.26 is low, hence acidosis.

Step 2: PCO_2 65 mm Hg is higher than normal (40 mm Hg), hence respiratory acidosis.

Step 3: Patient was managed with ventilatory support

Expected HCO_3 is 27 (1 meq increase for 10 mm hg increase in PCO_2), obtained HCO_3 is 22 meq/L, which is less than expected value - Suggesting coexistant metabolic acidosis.

Step 4: Find out the expected decrease in pH

(0.008 × increase in pCO_2): 25 × 0.008 = 0.2, 7.4 – 0.2 = 7.2. Here pH is 7.26 more than expected also suggests coexistant metabolic alkalosis.

Step 5: Interpret PaO_2 always in relation to FiO_2: patient on 60% O_2 PaO_2/FiO_2 = 60/0.6 =100, indicates acute respiratory distress syndrome.

Step 6: Find out A - aO_2 difference

PAO_2 = (760 – 47) × 0.6 – (65/0.8) – 60 = 379,

A – ao_2 = 346 – 60 = 286 mm Hg

The patient has respiratory acidosis and is hypoxic (PO_2/FiO_2 ratio 100). Pressure support is the mode of ventilation. Here the patient initiates and terminates each breath, tachypnea could be due to hypercarbia, hypoxia, pain or inadequate sedation. Hypercarbia indicates hypoventilation (since PCO_2 is inversely proportional to alveolar minute ventilation), so increasing the tidal volume should help.

In this very sick patient, a controlled mode of ventilation such as volume control or pressure control would be more appropriate until the hypoxia improves. One has to look for and correct airway obstruction, atelectasis or consolidation as possible causes for hypoxia.

Pulmonary Thromboembolism

The most common gas exchange abnormalities are hypoxemia (decreased arterial PO_2) and an increased alveolar-arterial O_2 tension gradient. Pathophysiological abnormalities are:

1. *Anatomic dead space increases* because breathed gas does not enter gas exchange units of the lung.
2. *Physiologic dead space increases* because ventilation to gas exchange units exceeds venous blood flow through the pulmonary capillaries.
3. *Increased pulmonary vascular resistance* due to vascular obstruction or platelet secretion of vasoconstricting neurohumoral agents such as serotonin. Release of vasoactive mediators can produce ventilation-perfusion mismatching at sites remote from the embolus, thereby accounting for a potential discordance between a small PE and a large alveolar-arterial O_2 gradient.
4. *Impaired gas exchange* due to increased alveolar dead space from vascular obstruction, hypoxemia from alveolar hypoventilation relative to perfusion in the non-obstructed lung, right-to-left shunting, and impaired carbon monoxide transfer due to loss of gas exchange surface.
5. *Alveolar hyperventilation* due to reflex stimulation of irritant receptors.
6. *Increased airway resistance* due to constriction of airways distal to the bronchi.
7. *Decreased pulmonary compliance* due to lung edema, lung hemorrhage, or loss of surfactant.

Case History 2

A 45-year-old man with a history of binge alcoholism is admitted with abdominal pain and vomiting of 2 days duration.

He is now in respiratory distress. On examination, blood pressure is 96/50, pulse 112/min, breaths 28/min, temperature 38.5° C, SpO_2 92%. The abdomen is distended and diffusely tender with no rebound tenderness and no bowel sounds are heard. A chest X-ray shows a small left pleural effusion and bilateral diffuse infiltrates. Differential diagnosis
• Acute pancreatitis is the most possible diagnosis.
• A perforated hollow viscus with secondary peritonitis
• Spontaneous bacterial peritonitis
    Abdominal imaging with ultrasound and CT reveal a grossly enlarged pancreas with patchy areas of decreased contrast uptake. There are small amounts of fluid within the peritoneal and left pleural cavities

Investigations

Hb 15.5 g/dL	WBC 14400/mm³	blood glucose 200	bilirubin 1.5
creatinine 1.5	calcium 8 (all mg/dL)	amylase 300 IU/mL	lipase 1400 IU/mL
pH 7.41	PCO₂ 31	HCO₃ 21	PO₂ 59

Interpretation of ABG

Step 1: pH 7.41 is in normal range, indicate normal acid-base status or a mixed acid base disorder.

Step 2: PCO_2 31 mm Hg is lower than normal, hence respiratory alkalosis.

Step 3: Expected HCO_3 is 22 (2 meq decrease for every 10 mm Hg decrease in PCO_2), obtained HCO_3 is 21 meq/L, less than expected value—coexistant metabolic acidosis.

Step 4: Find out the expected increase in pH (0.008 × decrease in PCO_2), 9 × 0.008 = 0.072 7.4 + 0.072 = 7.472, Here pH is 7.41 - less than expected also suggests coexistant metabolic acidosis.

Step 5: Interpret PaO_2, always in relation to FiO_2, Patient on 40% O_2 PaO_2/FiO_2 = 59/0.40 = 148, indicating acute respiratory distress syndrome.

Step 6: Find out A - aO_2 difference
PaO_2 = (760 – 47) × 0.4 – (31/0.8) – 59 = 379, A – aO_2 = 260 – 59 = 201 mm Hg.

The patient has a high alveolar-arterial O_2 difference of 20 mm Hg. The PaO_2/FiO_2 ratio is 147.5 which along with the X-ray picture of bilateral lung infiltrates suggests a diagnosis of acute respiratory distress syndrome (ARDS). He will require mechanical ventilation.

How would you handle the dyspnea and impaired oxygenation? The oxygen saturation picks up to 94% with 40% oxygen given by facemask.

On his way, back from radiology the patient becomes increasingly distressed, agitated and sits up on the trolley. The pulse oximeter reading intermittently falls to 75%. He is shifted to ICU and the ABGs repeated:

pH 7.30   PCO₂ 46   PO₂ 5 2   HCO₃ 20

Interpret the blood gas values interpretation of ABG

Step 1: pH 7.3 is low, hence acidosis.

Step 2: PCO_2 46 mm Hg is higher than normal 40 mm Hg, hence respiratory acidosis.

Step 3: Expected HCO_3 is 24.5 (1 meq increase for every 10 mm Hg increase in PCO_2), obtained HCO_3 is 20 meq/L, less than expected value—coexistent metabolic acidosis.

Step 4: Find out the expected decrease in pH (0.008 × increase in PCO_2): $6 \times 0.008 = 0.048$ $7.4 - 0.048 = 7.352$, Here pH is 7.30 less than expected also suggests coexistent metabolic acidosis.

Step 5: Interpret PaO_2, always in relation to FiO_2, Patient on 40% O_2 $PaO_2/FiO_2 = 52/0.40 = 130$ indicating acute respiratory distress syndrome

Step 6: Find out A - aO_2 difference

$PAO_2 = (760 - 47) \times 0.4 - 46/0.8) - 58 = 380$, A – $aO_2 = 260 - 52 = 208$ mm Hg

Both sets of values show hypoxia which is worse in the second measurement. Hypoxia leads to hyperventilation and a low PCO_2 in the first reading. In the second measurement, there is acidosis which is partly respiratory (PCO_2 46) and partly metabolic (HCO_3 20). The increases in PCO_2 and PO_2 indicate the patient has impending respiratory failure and the metabolic component of the acidosis could be due to lactate accumulation due to sepsis. *The patient is intubated and ventilated. He require vasopressors, antibiotics, enteral feeding and made a gradual recovery over three weeks.*

Case History 3

A 12-year-old girl is brought to casualty in severe breathlessness. She is sweating, tachypneic, tachycardic and cyanosed. Examination shows prolonged expiration and wheezes audible all over both lungs. Oxygen saturation is 80% but picks up rapidly to 98% on being given 4 liters of oxygen by facemask. However, when the mask is removed she rapidly desaturates to 90%.

Why is this patient's SpO_2 so dependent on inhaled oxygen? It is obvious that all the oxygen being breathed in is not getting to the blood. The patient requires a high inspired oxygen to maintain her arterial oxygenation. What is the arterial oxygen tension?

Investigations - ABG

pH 7.48   PCO$_2$ 30 mm Hg   PO$_2$ 58   HCO$_3$ 23
(while breathing 28% oxygen)

Interpretation of ABG

Step 1: pH 7.48 is in high, hence alkalosis.

Step 2: PCO_2 30 mm Hg is lower than normal 40 mm Hg, hence respiratory alkalosis.

Step 3: Expected HCO_3 is 22 (2 meq decrease for every 10 mm Hg decrease in PCO_2), obtained HCO_3 is 23 meq/L, almost identical – acute respiratory alkalosis.

Step 4: Find out the expected increase in pH ($0.008 \times$ decrease in PCO_2): $10 \times 0.008 = 0.08$ $7.4 + 0.08 = 7.48$, Here the obtained value is 7.48 simple respiratory alkalosis

Step 5: Interpret PaO_2 always in relation to FiO_2 patient on 28% O_2 $PaO_2/FiO_2 = 58/0.28 = 207$ indicating defective oxygenation.

ARDS is possible if there are bilateral lung infiltrates.

Step 6: Find out A - aO_2 difference

$PAO_2 = (760 - 47) \times 0.28 - (30/0.8) - 58 = 162$, A – $aO_2 = 162 - 58 = 104$ mm Hg.

Asthma causes airway obstruction due to bronchoconstriction and mucosal edema, leading to air trapping and alveolar hyperinflation. Hypoxemia and hypocapnia ensue. Calculation of the alveolar-arterial oxygen difference allows quantification of the defect in oxygenation which can occur in asthma and all other lung diseases that cause hypoxia.

Why does she have a low PCO₂?

Asthmatics hyperventilate unless they have developed respiratory failure and carbon dioxide tension is inversely proportional to alveolar minute ventilation.

If this patient develops respiratory failure how would she be managed?

She would need to be subjected to tracheal intubation and mechanical ventilation until the acute worsening of bronchial constriction and inflammatory airway narrowing subsides.

How would you ventilate a patient with severe asthma in respiratory failure?

A volume controlled mode would be preferable to pressure control to provide an assured minute volume. A long expiratory time is needed to allow complete expiration and reduce air trapping and dynamic hyperventilation. Higher than usual airway pressures may be tolerated as the narrow airways prevent the high pressure reaching the alveoli thereby preventing barotrauma.

Case History 4

A 35-year-old female on maintenance hemodialysis for endstage renal failure secondary to chronic glomerulonephritis is admitted with a 3-day history of fever, cough and breathlessness. She was dialyzed the previous day. BP is 180/100 mmHg, pulse 120/min, respiratory rate 30/min, SPO$_2$ 94%. There is a pedal edema and crackles audible over both lungs. Cardiac examination is normal.

Investigations - ABG

pH27   PCO$_2$ 58   PO$_2$ 79   HCO$_3$ 26   ABE -2

Interpret These Values

Step 1: pH 7.27 is low pH 7.45, hence acidosis

Step 2: PCO$_2$ 58 mm Hg is high, hence respiratory acidosis

Step 3: Expected HCO$_3$ is 26 (1 meq increase for 10 mm hg increase in PCO$_2$), obtained HCO$_3$ is 26 meq/L, hence simple respiratory acidosis

Step 4: Find out the expected decrease in pH (0.008 × increase in PCO$_2$):

18 × 0.008 = 0. 144.7.4 – 0.144 = 7.256. Here the obtained pH is identical to obtained pH, hence simple respiratory acidosis

Step 5: Interpret PaO$_2$, always in relation to FiO$_2$, patient on room air - FiO$_2$ 0.21, PaO$_2$/FiO$_2$79/0.21 = 390 (normal).

Step 6: Find out A - aO$_2$ difference PAO$_2$ = (760 – 47) × 0.21 – (58/0.8) = 150 – 79 = 71= 379, A – aO$_2$ = 379 – 47 = 332 mm Hg.

What is your analysis of the situation?

There is an acute respiratory acidosis: low pH, high PCO$_2$, indicates that the acidosis is respiratory and there is hardly any compensation (bicarbonate rise by 2 from 24 to 26 mmol/L closely corresponds to near 20 mm Hg rise in PCO$_2$) indicating it is acute. The normal base excess indicates there is no metabolic component. This is unlikely in a patient with renal failure. This could be due to the fact that she has been dialyzed recently.

Over the course of the day she becomes increasingly dyspneic. A chest radiograph shows bilateral lower zone patchy opacities and cardiac enlargement. This was interpreted as indicating fluid overload and she underwent further hemodialysis with removal of 4 liters of fluid. The dyspnea worsened, SpO$_2$ fell to 80% despite high flow oxygen, and repeat ABGs showed:

pH 7.30   PCO$_2$ 49   PO$_2$ 55   HCO$_3$ 25   ABE 0

On 80% O$_2$

What is the Situation?

Step 1: pH 7.30 is low pH 7.45, hence acidosis
Step 2: PCO_2 49 mm Hg is high hence respiratory acidosis
Step 3: Expected HCO_3 is 25 (1 meq increase for 10 mm Hg increase in PCO_2), obtained HCO_3 is 25 meq/L,
hence simple respiratory acidosis
Step 4: Find out the expected decrease in pH ($0.008 \times$ increase in PCO_2): $9 \times 0.008 = 0.072$. $7.4 - 0.072 = 7.328$
Since the obtained pH is almost identical to obtained pH, diagnosis is simple respiratory acidosis
Step 5: Interpret PaO_2 always in relation to FiO_2: patient on room air - FiO_2 0.21, PaO_2/FiO_2 55/0.80 = 70 diagnostic of ARDS.
Step 6: Find out A – aO_2 difference
$PAO_2 = (760 - 47) \times 0.80 - (55/0.8) = 560 - 70 = 490$, A – aO_2 = 490 – 55 = 445 mm Hg.

There is severe hypoxemia and respiratory acidosis. The bilateral pulmonary opacities persisted even after ultrafiltration and the PaO_2/FiO_2 ratio was 200 mm Hg, so the probable diagnosis is the acute respiratory distress syndrome.

She is placed on noninvasive ventilatory support through a tight fitting facemask. There is an initial improvement in SPO_2 to 92% on a FiO_2 of 60% with expiratory pressure set at 5 and inspiratory pressure at 12 cm H_2O. However, she is unable to tolerate the mask and is intubated for controlled mechanical ventilation.

What are the Indications for Noninvasive Ventilation?

Noninvasive ventilation (NIV) is used to avoid the complications of intubation in those patients who do not need full mechanical ventilation. The patients must be conscious and able to cooperate by tolerating the mask. The two main indications for NIV are respiratory failure due to acute exacerbations of chronic obstructive lung disease and cardiogenic pulmonary edema. In states of hypoxic respiratory failure such as ARDS, NIV may delay the need for intubation but this is often eventually needed. It can also be useful in weaning patients off mechanical ventilation, in the obesity-hypoventilation syndrome, chest wall injuries and postoperative patients.

> The chest X-ray taken after intubation and initiation of mechanical ventilation shows opacities affecting middle and lower zones of both lungs. PaO_2 remains below 60 mm Hg on 90% oxygen. How should this patient be ventilated?

High PEEP, low tidal volume, pressure controlled ventilation is indicated. The ARDS net study recommends: Tidal volume 6 mL/kg ideal body weight, FiO_2 to maintain saturation of 85–90% with a goal of reducing FiO_2 to below 0.6, PEEP (titrated to the FiO_2) upto 18–20 cm H_2O, and plateau inspiratory pressure below 30 cm H_2O. These measures limit ventilator induced lung injury (barotrauma due to high inflation pressures and volutrauma due to overdistension of normal parts of lung, VILI.

> She is ventilated on a lung protection strategy using a tidal volume of 6 mL/kg, PEEP 16 and plateau pressure was limited to 28 cm H_2O. The oxygen saturation remains at 80–82% despite 100% inspired oxygen. What can we do to improve oxygenation?

Refractory hypoxemia in ARDS can be treated by several manoeuvres. Inhaled nitric oxide has been used to improve blood flow to relatively better ventilated parts of lung but has shown no improvement in mortality. Decreasing the inspiratory time (inverse ratio) improves oxygenation but may cause overdistension and VILI. Prone positioning improves oxygenation by improving the distribution of pulmonary blood flow and recruiting dependent areas of lung. Finally, newer modes of lung support such as high frequency oscillation and extracorporeal membrane oxygenation may be used.

> The patient was turned prone and with the same ventilator settings SPO_2 improved to 88%. She was maintained in the prone position for 16 hours and then turned to supine and lateral positions. Over the next 2 days the inspired O_2 concentration was reduced to 60%. PEEP was then gradually reduced and she could be extubated 5 days later.

Case History 5

A 60-year-old chronic smoker is admitted with a one week history of fever, cough and drowsiness. He is centrally cyanosed with an oxygen saturation of 65%. Chest X-ray shows over inflation and bronchiectatic cavities in both mid zones. He is administered oxygen and antibiotics and the SPO_2 rises to 92%. *ABGs on 40% O_2*: pH 7.29 PCO_2 72 PO_2 58 HCO_3 32

What is the Acid-Base Disorder?

Step 1: pH 7.2930 is low, hence acidosis
Step 2: PCO_2 72 mm Hg is high, hence respiratory acidosis,
Step 3: H/o smoking and X-ray suggestive of chronic lung disaese expected HCO_3 is 36 (4 meq increase for 10 mm hg increase in PCO_2), obtained HCO_3 is 32 meq/L, hence respiratory acidosis with metabolic acidosis or acute respiratory acidosis with chronic respiratory acidosis.
Step 4: Find out the expected decrease in pH (0.003 × increase in PCO_2): 32 × 0.003 = 0. 096. 7.4 – 0.096 = 7.304. Here the obtained pH is almost identical to obtained pH.
Step 5: Interpret PaO_2, always in relation to FiO_2, patient on room air - FiO_2 0.21, PaO_2/FiO_2 58/0.40 = 145 diagnostic of ARDS.
Step 6: Find out A - AO_2 difference
   $PAO_2 = (760 – 47) × 0.40 – (72/0.8) = 286 – 90 = 196$, A – aO_2 = 196 – 58 = 148 mm Hg.

Despite additional oxygen the patient appeared increasingly breathless. He was started on noninvasive ventilation by face mask. On an inspired oxygen concentration of 35%, the SPO_2 improved 97%. The patient tolerated the mask, his respiratory rate decreased and he appeared settled.

ABG values on the next day:
pH 7.48 PCO_2 48 PO_2 70 HCO_3 35

What is the Acid-Base Disorder?

Step 1: pH 7.48 is low, hence alkalosis
Step 2: PCO_2 48 mm Hg is high, suggestive of metabolic alkalosis
Step 3: HCO_3 is 35 mmol/L, Expected PCO_2 is 40 + (0.7 × 11) = 47.7 Suggests *simple metabolic alkalosis*

What is the Explanation for Metabolic Alkalosis?

There is a gratifying decrease in carbon dioxide tension and improvement in oxygenation. The HCO_3 has increased in spite of the fall in PCO_2 leading to a metabolic alkalosis. This could be due to

- Hypochloremia and hypokalemia from diuresis (was he on a loop diuretic?)
- Post-hypercapnic metabolic alkalosis.

The patient was not on a diuretic and there was no cardiac failure or edema.

The cause is **post-hypercapnic metabolic alkalosis.**

Because of chronic hypercapnia, renal compensation caused a raised HCO_3 to help bring the pH towards normal. The increased ventilation (by NIV) has reduced the PCO_2 but HCO_3 remains high because renal readjustment takes several days. This metabolic alkalosis is clinically relevent because it can induce hypoventilation sufficient to cause hypoxia. Treatment consists of cautious saline administration to correct any hypovolemia, correction of hypokalemia if present and the use of a carbonic anhydrase inhibitor such as acetazolamide. The patient was treated with acetazolamide 125 mg twice daily and was taken off noninvasive ventilation the next day. He remained mildly hypercapnic and hypoxic but was less dyspneic, afebrile and the pH came down to 7.33.

Section 3

Metabolic Acid-Base Abnormalities

Maintenance of H⁺ Ion Balance

A Vimala

OVERVIEW

Tight control of H^+ ions is of great importance for maintaining cell function. H^+ ions bind avidly to proteins and make them cat ionic. This will change the shape and function of the cells. Around 70,000,000 nmoles of H^+ ions are formed and consumed daily. Normal ECF H^+ ion concentration is maintained at a low level of 40 nmol/L. This is due to very effective buffering mechanism and also by elimination of CO_2 and nitrogenous wastes.

MAINTENANCE OF H⁺ ION BALANCE

There are three important primary mechanisms which regulate H^+ ion concentration and prevent the development of acidosis or alkalosis. The first line of defense is by chemical buffering which is immediate. This is followed by respiratory compensation which is fast. Renal adjustment is the third important mechanism and is slow.

1. The chemical acid-base buffer system.
2. The respiratory center that regulates the removal of CO_2 and thus changes H_2CO_3 in ECF.
3. The kidneys which can excrete either acid or alkaline urine and thus regulate H^+ ion concentration.

Buffering of H⁺ Ions in the Body

Chemical Buffering

This is the immediate first line of defense. Chemical buffers cannot remove or add H⁺ ions from or to body fluids. They keep H⁺ ion in the bound state and regulate free H⁺ ion concentration in plasma till a new balance is established. A buffer can reversibly bind H⁺ ions

H⁺ + Buffer ↔ buffer.

When H⁺ ion concentration increases, H⁺ will bind to the buffer which remains in the undissociated state forming a weak acid. When H⁺ ion concentration decreases, H⁺ buffer will dissociate to H⁺ and buffer. Buffering of H⁺ ions will continue as long as the buffers are present. There are three important buffer systems.

Respiratory Mechanism

Chemical buffering is followed by respiratory changes. The newly formed H_2CO_3 is a weak acid and hence will dissociate immediately into CO_2 and H_2O. The CO_2 is eliminated by increasing the rate of respiration.

Renal Mechanism

The third important mechanism is by the kidney. Compensation is complete and kidneys play a pivotal role in acid base regulation. This is mainly by the regulation of HCO_3 concentration and secretion of H⁺ ions.

Chemical Buffering

In chemical buffering, immediate protection is by buffers.

Buffers

A buffer system consists of a weak acid/alkali combination which resists any change in pH by changing the relative concentrations of its own acid and alkali. There are many buffer systems in body fluids.

1. Bicarbonate buffer system (carbonic acid/bicarbonate).
2. Phosphate buffer system (HPO_4/H_2PO_4).
3. Large proteins such as albumin, hemoglobin and bone buffers. Large proteins carry many amino and carboxyl groups which can act as proton donors and acceptors. *Bone is an important buffer in chronic metabolic acidosis.*
4. NH_4 buffer system.

Bicarbonate Buffer System (BBS)

The buffer system has two components:
1. Weak acid – H_2CO_3 (carbonic acid)
2. Weak base – $NaHCO_3$ (sodium bicarbonate).

H_2CO_3 is formed in the body fluids by the combination of CO_2 and H_2O. This is a slow reaction. The speed of the reaction is increased by carbonic anhydrase enzyme present in the pulmonary alveoli and renal tubular epithelial cells. The second component occurs when $NaHCO_3$ readily dissociates to Na^+ and HCO_3^-. When a strong acid like HCl is added, H^+ ions combine with HCO_3^- to form very weak H_2CO_3. The excess carbon dioxide is removed by lungs.

$$H^+ + HCO_3 \rightarrow H_2CO_3 \rightarrow H_2O + CO_2.$$

Similarly, when a strong alkali like Na OH is added

$$NaOH + H_2CO_3 \rightarrow Na\ HCO_3$$

The weak base Na HCO_3 replaces the strong alkali Na OH. This leads to reduction in H_2CO_3 and this will be replaced by CO_2 reacting with H_2O.

The decreasing CO_2 will reduce the rate of respiration and CO_2 will increase. The bicarbonate concentration is regulated by the kidney. Bicarbonate buffer system (BBS) is the most important extracellular buffer. The buffer capacity of the buffer will depend on quantity and dissociation constant of the buffer. BBS is low in its quantity and dissociation constant is 6.1 away from the pH of ECF 7.4. The two elements of the BBS HCO_3 and CO_2 can be tightly regulated by kidneys and lungs respectively. Hence this is the most important buffer system in ECF.

The Phosphate Buffer System

This is the major buffer in ICF and renal tubular fluid. In ECF, it's buffering bower is low as the concentration is only 8% of BBS. In renal tubular fluid phosphates are concentrated. pH is lower than the ECF pH. This is closer to the dissociation constant of the buffer system which is 6.8. In ICF, the concentration is high and pH is close to 6.8. Hence this is a very important buffer system.

$HCl + Na_2 HPO_4 \rightarrow Na H_2PO_4 + Na Cl.$

$Na OH + Na H_2PO_4 \rightarrow Na_2 HPO_4 + H_2O$

Protein Buffer System

They are very important ICF buffers. All cell membranes except RBC membrane permit only a small amount of diffusion of H^+ ions and HCO_3. This is a slow process. In RBCs there is a rapid equilibrium.

$Hb + H^+ \rightarrow H Hb.$

High concentration of proteins inside the cells and the dissociation constant which is very close to the pH 7.35 makes it a very effective intracellular buffer. 60–70% of chemical buffering occurs within the cells.

RESPIRATORY CONTROL OF ACID-BASE BALANCE

This is the second line of defense and the control is by regulating pCO_2 by lungs. Elimination of CO_2 by lungs balances the metabolic formation of CO_2. Inside the cells CO_2 is produced from metabolic processes. CO_2 diffuses into the interstitial fluid and blood. It reaches the pulmonary venous blood and diffuses into the alveoli and is transferred to the atmosphere by pulmonary ventilation. Dissolved CO_2 in ECF is 1.2 millimoles/L which corresponds to $PaCO_2$ of 40 mm of Hg. If the metabolic production of CO_2 increases the rate of respiration will increase and vice versa. If the rate of formation of CO_2 is constant, the only factor that can influence PCO_2 is rate of ventilation. Increasing the rate of ventilation to twice normal, ECF pH will increase by 0.23. i.e. from 7.4 to 7.63.

Similarly, reducing the rate of respiration to one fourth of normal the pH will reduce by 0.45, i.e. from 7.4 to 6.95. When pH increases and rate of respiration decrease the O_2 delivered to the blood will also decrease. Reduction in PO_2 has a stimulatory effect on respiratory center. This prevents further reduction in respiratory rate, hence the compensation will not be complete.

RENAL REGULATION OF ACID-BASE BALANCE

Kidneys controls acid base balance by tightly regulating the H$^+$ ion concentration in blood. This is by excreting an acidic urine when H$^+$ ions increase or excreting HCO_3^- ions when H$^+$ ions decrease.

Production of H$^+$ Ions

H$^+$ ions are released when proteins are metabolized and when fruits and vegetables rich in K$^+$ are consumed. H$^+$ ions are also removed by organic acids as K$^+$ salts. About 80 m Eq of non-volatile acids are produced daily. These nonvolatile acids cannot be excreted by lungs and are excreted by the kidneys. Kidneys also have to conserve and generate new HCO_3 under normal conditions.

Renal Handling of HCO_3 (Fig. 14.1)

The processes involved are glomerular filtration, reabsorption and regeneration of HCO_3.

Normally, about 180 Liters of plasma is filtered and quantity of HCO_3 filtered is 25 × 180 = 4500 mmol/day.

Bicarbonate is completely filtered by the glomeruli.

Renal handling of HCO_3

Site	mmol/day
Glomerular filtration	4500
Tubular reabsorption	
Proximal	4000
Loop	400
Distal	100

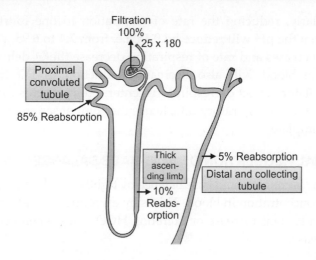

Fig. 14.1: Renal handling of bicarbonate

Plasma concentration of bicarbonate is 25 mm Eq/L. Daily about 4500 mEq of bicarbonate is filtered in a person who has a glomerular filtrate of 180 liters daily. 85–90% (4000 mEq) of filtered bicarbonate is normally reabsorbed in the proximal tubule, 10% (400 mEq) in the thick ascending limb of loop of Henle and around 5% (100 mEq) in the distal and collecting tubule. Normal urine contains **no bicarbonate.**

PHYSIOLOGY OF HCO$_3^-$ REABSORPTION AND H$^+$ IONS SECRETION

Bicarbonate reabsorption occurs in all segments of the nephron except thin descending limb and thin ascending limb of loop of Henle.

Reabsorption in Proximal Tubules (Fig. 14.2)

This is the main site of reabsorption of HCO$_3^-$ as 80% of the filtered HCO$_3^-$ is reabsorbed here and is linked with the removal of equal number of H$^+$ ions. So there is no net change in acid-base status. The process starts with the formation of CO$_2$ inside the cell or diffusion of CO$_2$ from the lumen to the

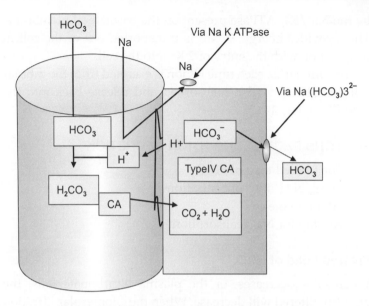

Fig. 14.2: Reaborption of bicarbonate in proximal tubule

cell. Carbonic anhydrase type II is present inside the cells. CO_2 will combine with H_2O to form H_2CO_3 which will dissociate into H^+ and HCO_3^-. The HCO_3^- that is formed will exit along the basolateral membrane into the interstitial fluid and to the peritubular capillary blood. H^+ ions that is formed inside the cell is excreted in to the lumen via Na^+ H^+ antiporter. This protein transporter is present in the luminal border of the cell membrane. Na^+ also will combine with the carrier protein. H^+ will bind to the other side of the carrier protein. Thus H^+ will be secreted into the lumen and Na^+ will be reabsorbed. The secreted H^+ ion will combine with HCO_3^- that is filtered by the glomeruli to form H_2CO_3. Carbonic anhydrase enzyme type IV is present in the proximal tubular lumen. In presence of the enzyme, H_2CO_3 that is formed dissociates rapidly into H_2O and CO_2. CO_2 will diffuse into the cell.

The entry of Na from the lumen to the cell is along the concentration gradient. The intracellular sodium is kept low by the $Na^+/K^+/ATPase$ present on the basolateral membrane. This provides energy. 3 Na^+ is transported out of the cell in conjunction with the entry of 2 K^+ into the cell.

To summarize each time H^+ ion is excreted from the tubular cell one HCO_3^- is also reabsorbed and release back into the blood (Ref: Fig. 14.2).

FACTORS REGULATING H⁺ ION SECRETION

1. The filtered load of HCO_3^-
2. Luminal H^+ ion concentration
3. H^+ ion in the cell
4. Avidity for Na^+ reabsorption.

Filtered Load of HCO_3^-

When GFR decreases, or the plasma bicarbonate falls, the quantity filtered will decrease. When the Glomerular filtration decreases from 180 to 100 liters the filtered load of bicarbonate will be 25 × 100 = 2500 mmoles instead of 25 × 180 = 4500 mmoles. If the plasma concentration of bicarbonate decreases from 25 to 10 mmoles/L, the filtered load of HCO_3 will decrease from the normal filtered load of 4500 mmoles to 1800 mmoles/day (180 × 10). Since H^+ ions have no other acceptors, H^+ ion secretion also will drop by 50%.

Luminal H⁺ Ion Concentration

If the luminal H^+ ion concentration increases rapidly, this will limit further secretion of H^+ ions. If formation of H_2CO_3 is delayed by drugs like carbonic anhydrase inhibitors, luminal H^+ ions will increase and prevent further secretion of H^+ ions. This will prevent reabsorption of HCO_3.

H⁺ Ion in the Cell

Increase in the intracellular H^+ ions can activate the $Na^+ H^+$ antiporter and increase the secretion of H^+ ions. This effect is limited because the availability of HCO_3 is less in conditions associated with metabolic acidosis.

Avidity for Na⁺ Reabsorption

When there is ECF volume expansion as with $NaHCO_3$ infusions there is an inhibition for reabsorption of HCO_3^- thus there will be failure to increase the H⁺ ion secretion.

In ECF volume contraction with increase in Na reabsorption there is increase in H⁺ ion secretion. This is mediated through RAAS system.

SECRETION OF H⁺ IONS FROM THE INTERCALATED CELLS OF DISTAL TUBULE AND COLLECTING TUBULE

H⁺ ions are secreted by primary active transport. Inside the cell CO_2 will combine with water to form H_2CO_3 which will dissociate into HCO_3^- and H⁺ ions. HCO_3^- is released back to the blood. H⁺ ions are secreted actively by the H⁺ ATPase pump into the tubular lumen. Only 5% of the H⁺ ion secretion occurs in this segment but this is very important because H⁺ ion secretions can increase by 900 fold in the collecting tubules and pH of the tubular fluid is lowered to 4.5.

HCO₃ Reabsorption in the Collecting Ducts

1. The amount of HCO_3^- reabsorbed is much *smaller* than in the proximal tubule.
2. Reabsorption can be easily *saturated* by increase in HCO_3^- load (low V_{max}).
3. Can occur with *larger transepithelial pH difference* (4.5–7.4) than in the proximal tubules (6.8–7.4).
4. This is *not mediated by luminal carbonic anhydrase.*
5. *H⁺ ion secretion is mostly by luminal proton and by proton- K⁺ ATPases* of alpha-intercalated cells.
6. *Basolateral transport* of HCO_3^- is via Cl⁻ *exchangers.*
7. Beta-intercalated cells secrete bicarbonate into the lumen and extrude H⁺ into the ECF.

Regulation: HCO_3 reabsorption in the collecting duct is stimulated by the following:

1. *High concentration of H^+ inside collective duct* activate the H^+ pumps in the cells (as in acidosis or K^+ deficiency).
2. Respiratory or metabolic acidosis, *more proton pumps* are inserted into the luminal membrane of alpha-intercalated cells.
3. Low [H^+] (i.e. at more *alkaline pH) in the tubular fluid.*
4. Increase in the *negativity of the tubular lumen* when Na^+ reabsorption by principal cells is increased by *aldosterone* or when the *load of slowly reabsorbed* PO_4^-, SO_4^- or HCO_3^- increase.
5. *Aldosterone* acts directly to increase H^+ secreting pumps in alpha intercalated cells.

RENAL PRODUCTION OF HCO_3

When excess of H^+ ions are secreted into tubular fluid they have to be buffered inside the lumen. This is because the luminal pH can be lowered only to 4.5. This corresponds to H^+ ions concentration of 0.03 Eq/L. Daily around 80 mEq of non-volatile acids have to be excreted and this would require around 2667 liters of urine if H^+ ions are to be secreted freely, maintaining the pH at 4.5. The most important buffers in the tubular lumen are NH_4 buffer system and phosphate buffer system.

NH_4^+ Excretion (Fig. 14.3)

Renal production of ammonium. Glutamine a neutral compound is derived from dietary and endogenous proteins. Glutamine is actively transported into cells of proximal, distal and collecting tubule from the peritubular capillary blood and from the filtrate. Within the cell, glutamine enters the mitochondria and is deamidated by glutaminase I enzyme and deaminated by glutamic dehydrogenase. This will result in two molecules of NH_4^+ and one of divalent alpha-ketoglutarate anion. This anion is oxidized to $2\ HCO_3^- + 4\ CO_2 + H_2O$. NH_4^+ is secreted into the

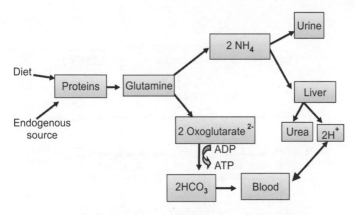

Fig. 14.3: Generation of new bicarbonate and NH_4 excretion

lumen through the Na^+-H^+ or NH_4^+ exchanger. Bicarbonate exits through basolateral cotransport with Na^+. For each NH_4^+ excreted, one new bicarbonate enters the ECF (Fig. 14.4).

Collecting tubule cell is freely permeable to NH_3 and impermeable to NH_4. The NH_3 that is formed inside the cell diffuses into the lumen where it combines with H^+ to form NH_4. NH_4 combines with chloride that is filtered and is excreted as NH_4Cl.

Under normal conditions the amount of H^+ ions secreted by the NH_4 buffer account for 50% of the acid secreted and 50% of the HCO_3 generated. The most important mechanism of excreting the acid load is by increasing the NH_4 secretion.

Generation of High Ammonium (NH_4) in Medullary Interstitium (Fig. 14.4)

Four steps are required for the excretion of NH_4:
1. As discussed earlier, ammonium is produced in cortical proximal tubules.
2. This is secreted into the proximal tubular lumen mainly through Na^+/H^+ antiporter system replacing H^+.
3. Reabsorption of NH_4 in the thick ascending limb of loop of Henle is via the Na^+ K^+ 2 Cl^- cotransporter replacing K^+.

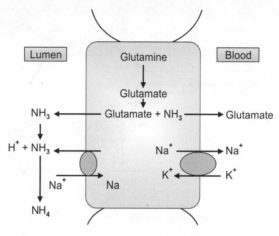

Fig. 14.4: Generation of NH_4

4. Secretion of NH_4 into the descending limb of loop of Henle and through the counter current system maintains high NH_4 in medullary interstitium. NH_4^+ dissociates into NH_3 (volatile) and H^+ ions. The gaseous NH_3 diffuses to the medullary interstitium and to the descending limb where the countercurrent system generates a corticomedullary NH_3 and NH_4^+ gradient. The NH_3 diffuses from the medullary interstitium to the acid fluid in the collecting duct where it reacts with H^+ forming impermeant NH_4^+ which is excreted in the urine.

Phosphate Buffer System in the Tubular Fluid (Fig. 14.5)

This buffer system is composed of HPO_4^- and H_2PO_4. This is a very effective buffer. There is relatively poor reabsorption of PO_4 from the tubule. Water is reabsorbed to a good extent. This will increase the concentration of the buffer. The dissociation constant of the buffer is 6.8 which is close to the pH of tubular fluid. This confers a very high buffer capacity. When excess of H^+ ions are secreted, this will combine with the HPO_4 that is filtered to form H_2PO_4. This H_2PO_4 will be excreted as Na Salt– NaH_2PO_4. CO_2 will combine with H_2O to form H_2CO_3 in the cell which dissociates

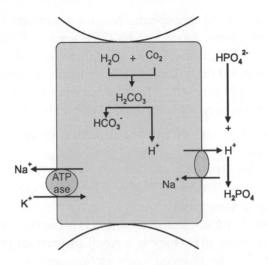

Fig. 14.5: Excretion of titratable acid

to H^+ and HCO_3^- inside the cell. The HCO_3 that is formed is a new molecule and not that is filtered. This new bicarbonate generation will replenish the depleted HCO_3 buffer.

Excretion of Titratable Acid

The major buffer in urine is phosphate. At pH 7.4 as in the glomerular filtrate, only 20% of the phosphate is in the di-acid phosphate form ($H_2PO_4^-$) and 80% is in the monoacid form (HPO_4^-).

In the *proximal tubule,* H^+ secretion progressively decrease pH to 6.8 and titrates up to 50% of the phosphate in the lumen to the diprotonated form $H_2PO_4^-$. Luminal Na^+ is reabsorbed in exchange for cell H^+ and exits, together with HCO_3^- formed in the cell across the basolateral membrane. For every proton secreted that titrates the phosphate in the lumen, there is generation of one molecule of bicarbonate that enters the circulation and helps to restore the buffering capacity of the body.

In the *collecting ducts* H^+ ion secretion, through luminal proton ATPases, can acidify the urine to pH < 6. At this pH practically all phosphate has been converted to the diprotonated form. Again, one HCO_3^- is generated for each H^+ secreted due to titration of the phosphate from the mono to the diprotonated form. Diprotonated phosphates are excreted. When urine pH is less than 5, other buffers such as creatinine and β-hydroxybutyrate contribute to titratable acid excretion

Regulation: The rate of urinary excretion of titratable acid depends on:

a. The *urine pH*
b. The *rate of excretion of buffers* (phosphate, creatinine and β-hydroxyburyrate).

In acidosis, titratable acid excretion is enhanced mostly due to the low urine pH. There is a small increase in phosphate excretion due to reduced reabsorption and loss of bone phosphate. β-hydroxybutyrate can contribute significantly up to 30% i.e. around 10 fold increment from 30 to 300 mmol/day of titratable acid excretion can occur in severe ketoacidosis when the urine pH is below 4.5.

The concentration of titratable acid (mEq/L) in the urine can be quantified by direct measurement.

Net Acid Excretion

To maintain acid-base homeostasis the non-volatile acids have to be excreted. To quantify this, the H^+ ions that are excreted in combination with non-bicarbonate buffers have to be measured. The important non-bicarbonate buffers as mentioned earlier are NH_4 and phosphates. The H^+ ion that is excreted as ammonium can be directly measured by measuring NH_4 in urine. The H^+ ions that are excreted in combination with PO_4 and to a very less extent with other organic acids can be quantified by measuring of the titratable acid. The normal pH of blood and thereby glomerular filtrate is 7.4. Urine is titrated with a strong alkali NAOH and the volume of NAOH required to titrate the urine pH back to 7.4 will give the H^+ secretion as PO_4. NAOH will not displace H^+ bound to NH_4.

Net Acid Excretion =

NH_4^+ excretion + (titratable acids excreted (in millie-quivalents) - the bicarbonate (mEq) in the urine.

The bicarbonate in urine is equal to the number of H^+ ions that are added to the blood.

SUMMARY OF BICARBONATE REABSORPTION AND REGENERATION

The kidney compensates for acid production by its ability to reclaim and regenerate bicarbonate. Bicarbonate filtered by glomeruli combines with a free proton secreted by the renal tubular cell to produce H_2CO_3. This is then converted by carbonic anhydrase to carbon dioxide which diffuses into the renal cell (along its concentration gradient). Inside the cell the pathway is reversed, with HCO_3 passing back into the blood and H^+ being secreted into the lumen to retrieve more bicarbonate. In addition, bicarbonate regeneration occurs because of carbon dioxide production within the tubular cell by cellular metabolism. The carbon dioxide is converted to H^+ and HCO_3^-. This HCO_3^- then diffuses into the blood, and the H^+ passes into the tubular lumen where it combines with an anion such as phosphate or ammonia and is excreted in the urine. This process produces new bicarbonate for buffering in the blood.

KEY POINTS

- To maintain H^+ ion balance H^+ ion production should be equal to H^+ ion excretion.
- Volatile acids are effectively buffered and CO_2 is regulated by adjusting ventilation.
- Non-volatile acids produced are handled by the kidney.
- Major site of bicarbonate reabsorption is proximal tubule.
- H^+ions in the distal tubule lumen and collecting tubule are mainly buffered by the phosphate buffers and NH_4.
- When H^+ ions increase due to extra-renal cause urinary NH_4 excretion increases to 500 fold to maintain H^+ ion balance.

15

Approach to Arterial Blood Gas Analysis

A Vimala

ABBREVIATIONS

ABG	Arterial blood gas
$AaDO_2$	Alveolar arterial oxygen gradient
AO_2	Alveolar oxygen partial pressure
BB	Buffer Base
BE	Base Excess
BE ecf	Base Excess in extracellular fluid
CH^+	Concentration of Hydrogen ion
CO_2	Carbon di oxide
FiO_2	Fraction of O_2 in inspired air
Hb	Hemoglobin
HCO_3	Bicarbonate
H_2CO_3	Carbonic acid
O_2CT	Oxygen content of blood
$PaCO_2$	Partial pressure of carbon dioxide in arterial blood
PaO_2	Partial pressure of oxygen in arterial blood
RQ	Respiratory quotient
Sat	Saturation
SBE	Standard base Excess
St HCO_3	Standard bicarbonate
T CO_2	Total carbon dioxide content of blood
THb	Total hemoglobin concentration
VBG	Venous blood gas

INTRODUCTION

ABG is an important tool to assess ventilation in critically ill patients. Venous blood gas (VBG) is helpful in assessing tissue perfusion. Though there are many values in the print out, blood gas analyzer measures only pH, PCO_2 and PO_2. All the other values are generated using the software in computer.

INDICATIONS AND TECHNIQUE OF COLLECTION OF SAMPLE

Indications for Blood Gas Analysis

1. *To assess acid base status of the patient*
   i. Patients with Multi Organ failure,
   ii. Acute Kidney Injury
   iii. Sepsis Syndrome
   iv. Cardiac Failure
   v. Suspected Hypoxic Encephalopathy
   vi. Renal tubular acidosis
   vii. Conditions that cause metabolic acidosis like Diabetes mellitus, Formic acid poisoning, Methyl alcohol etc.
2. *To assess oxygenation status.*

Technique of Collection of Sample

Blood sample should be collected very meticulously since any error in collection, storage or transport of sample to the laboratory can alter the blood gas values.

The basic procedure is a simple arterial puncture.

Sites of Puncture

- Radial artery — Is the most common site of puncture because of ease of access. The other arteries used for puncture are brachial artery and femoral artery
- In neonates umbilical artery is chosen for puncture.

   Radial artery puncture — Before puncturing radial artery "Allens" test should be performed to ensure that collateral blood supply is adequate from ulnar artery. If puncture of radial artery is difficult, femoral artery may be used. Needle is inserted at point of maximum pulsation just proximal to the proximal transverse skin crease at the wrist.

Brachial artery puncture — Needle is inserted medial to the biceps tendon over the point of maximum pulsation.

Femoral artery puncture — Introduce needle at mid inguinal point 2 cm below the inguinal ligament at point of maximum pulsation.

Central venous catheter sample — This sample is used for finding out mixed venous O_2 saturation in conditions like sepsis syndrome.

While drawing blood from peripheral vein for analysis, tourniquet should not be applied and artery should not be compressed.

Requirement for Drawing Blood

1. 1% plain lignocaine
2. 2 cc glass syringe
3. 23 G needle (blue) for radial and brachial artery puncture
4. 21 G needle (green) for femoral puncture
5. Rubber cap to seal needle
6. Heparin solution 1000 U/mL
7. Ice — for transport of sample to laboratory
8. Povidone iodine/spirit for cleaning
9. Gauze/cotton swab.

Procedure

1. Patient is made to lie supine. Puncture is done preferably in the non-dominant wrist resting on a saline bag extended to 20 to 30° angle.
2. Heparinize the syringe — draw about 0.1 mL of heparin into the syringe and flush well. Expel the heparin as heparin that sticks to the syringe is adequate for anticoagulation.
3. Identify the pulse lateral to the flexor carpi radialis tendon at the wrist and clean the area of puncture with spirit/povidone iodine.

4. Infiltrate minimal amount of lignocaine subcutaneously taking care to avoid a bulge that obscures palpation of the vessel.
5. Insert needle with bevel facing upwards at an angle of 20 to 30° to the horizontal.
6. Aspirate gently 1–2 mL of blood.
7. Withdraw needle and expel any air in the blood and syringe by gentle tapping and pushing the piston with needle up.
8. Quickly cap the needle with the rubber cap.
9. Label properly and put the needle in an ice bag.
10. Apply gauze/cotton swab and give firm pressure at the site of puncture for 5 minutes. Look for swelling or bleeding in which case pressure can should be continued.

To avoid errors, sample should be sent to the laboratory and analyzed within 20 to 30 minutes.

Precautions to be Followed While Collecting Blood Sample

1. Heparin is acidic and it will lower pH. Use heparin of lowstrength - 1000 U/ml. Syringe and needle are heparinized by drawing 0.5 ml of heparin into the syringe and is pushed through the needle. This will prevent dilution of blood sample with heparin.
2. Glass syringe should be used instead of plastic syringe as plastic syring is epermeable to air.
3. Syringe should be filled spontaneously.
4. Avoid air bubble inside the sample.

Transport of Sample

The sample should be processed immediately within 30 minutes. Blood is a living medium with continuous metabolism. Hence, cells will consume oxygen and produce CO_2. So delay in processing may lead to low PaO_2 and High PCO_2. To prevent this the sample should be stored in ice slush at 4°C. Sample should be shaken well before feeding into monitor. Avoid contact of blood with atmospheric air by putting a rubber cap over the needle and bending the needle.

Blood gas values in the arterial and venous sample is shown in Table 15.1.

Venus sample has a lower O_2, Higher PCO_2 and higher HCO_3 than arterial sample.

With changes in temperature, pH, PCO_2 and will change. The changes that occur when stored at 37° and 4° every 10 minutes is shown in Table 15.2. It is evident that significant changes occur when kept at 37°. If there is a delay in analysis the sample should be stored at 4°, to minimize the changes.

Normal ABG values in adult and neonates shown in Table 15.3.

Table 15.1: Comparison of blood gas analysis of arterial and venous samples

Parameters	Arterial	Venous
pH	Same	Same
PO_2	Higher	Lower
PCO_2	Lower	Higher
HCO_3	Lower	Higher

Table 15.2: Changes in ABG every 10 minutes (in stored sample)

Parameters	37°	4°
pH	0.01	0.001
PCO_2	0.1 mm Hg	0.01 mm Hg
PO_2	0.1 mm Hg	0.01 mm Hg

Table 15.3: Normal ABG values in adult and neonates

Parameters	Adult	Neonates
PH	7.35–7.45	7.35–7.40
PCO_2	35–45 mm Hg	35–45 mm Hg
PaO_2	98–100 mm Hg	50–70 mm Hg
HCO_3	22–25 mmol/L	20–24 mmol/L
Base excess	+2	+2

Explanation of Parameters in the ABG Printout

pH   log [H^+] in gram ions/L, P stands for "power index"
         pH is the negative logarithm of H^+ ion concentration

CH^+ Concentration of H^+ ions in nanomol/liter at 37°C

THb   Only few machines will measure Hb from the sample. So it is better to feed Hb value in the request since this is required to calculate the oxygen content.

Temperature—pH, PCO_2 and PO_2 are affected by temperature. Hence, patient's temperature has to be provided in the request. Otherwise, ABG machine will assume the temperature as 37°C and give the values.

BEecf, BB, BE

BB   Total buffer base. Normal value is 48–49 mmol/L

BE   Actual base excess in variance above or below BB 25% of BB is constituted by Hb, 50% by HCO_3 and 25% by proteins, phosphate, sulfate.

TCO_2 Sum of HCO_3 and CO_2

Standard HCO_3—This is the bicarbonate value for the given pH had the PCO_2 been 40 mm of Hg and temperature 37°C and is calculated using the Henderson's equation.

Example: If the pH is 7.3 at standard bicarbonate will be PCO_2 of 40 mm Hg and temperature of 37°C, standard HCO_3 will be 50 = 24 × 40/HCO_3 = 24 × 40/50 = 20

Actual Bicarbonate—This is calculated based on the measured PCO_2 and temperature.

Example: For a pH of 7.3 and PCO_2 60 mm of Hg actual bicarbonate will be 50 = 24 × 60/HCO_3 = 24 × 60/50 = 29

TCO_2—Is the sum of HCO_3 and amount of dissolved CO_2. For each mm of CO_2, 0.03 mL of CO_2 is dissolved per 100 mL. For a TCO_2 of 40 mm dissolved CO_2 will be 0.12.

Oxygen saturation—It is the % of Hb that is saturated with O_2.

(Respiratory quotient) (RQ)—Is calculated by dividing CO_2 liberated per minute ÷ O_2 utilized per minute.

Normal value is 200/2 = 100

FiO_2 — Is the fraction of O_2 in inspired air. FiO_2 in normal atmospheric air is 21%.

Oxygen saturation — This is the volume of O_2 that is combined with Hb.

This is usually measured by pulse oxymeter. The technique measures peripheral hemoglobin saturation (SaO_2).

Artifacts of measurements are:

- It is affected by high intensity light
- Fetal Hb when present > 50% can give an error in SaO_2
- Normal saturation is 95–98% clinical cyanosis become evident when saturation is < 75%. At a PO_2 of 40 mm Hg, 75% of Hb A is saturated.

Oxygen Content — It is the concentration of total O_2 in blood. Expressed as volume %. Patients with anemia may have normal saturation because of cardiac compensation but decreased oxygen content as Hb is less for transporting oxygen.

Oxygen Delivery

It is the product of arterial O_2 content and cardiac output. Hence, it is directly affected by changes in PaO_2, Hb concentration and cardiac output.

KEY POINTS

- Arterial blood sample is analyzed for assessment of ventilation and is a clue to diagnosis of pulmonary abnormalities.
- Proper collection technique is essential for accurate results.
- Delay in analysis of sample can give erroneous results.
- pH and PCO_2 are measured and HCO_3 is calculated by the computer.

Interpretation of Arterial Blood Gas

A Vimala, G Krishnakumar

OVERVIEW

The familiar Henderson-Hasselbalch equation is used to find out the pH resulting from the carbon dioxide dissociation equation.

The equation is

$$pH = pKa + \log (HCO_3/PCO_2 \times 0.03)$$

Henderson equation is the simplified form of the above equation and is shown below

$[H^+] = 24 \times PCO_2/HCO_3$ (hydrogen ion in nmol/L, PCO_2 in mm Hg, HCO_3 in mmol/L)

In simple terms, the Henderson-Hasselbalch equation states that the body's state of acidemia or alkalaemia can be expressed as the ratio between bicarbonate and carbon dioxide concentrations (This does not consider the contribution of the other buffer systems but is reasonably accurate for most clinical situations). Bicarbonate level is controlled mainly by the kidneys and carbon dioxide level by the lungs. There are four possible derangements:

1. Respiratory acidosis
2. Respiratory alkalosis
3. Metabolic acidosis
4. Metabolic alkalosis.

In respiratory acidosis and respiratory alkalosis, the rate of ventilation is the single factor determining carbon dioxide excretion.

Metabolic acid-base disorders are caused by addition of new anions other than bicarbonate, hence bicarbonate is not the single determining factor in deciding pH in metabolic abnormalities. For example in diabetic ketoacidosis (DKA) the primary acid-base defect is an accumulation of acid in the form of β butyric acid and acetooacetic acids. Changes in pH caused by disorders such as DKA reduce the [HCO_3] as a result of buffering and affect the HCO_3/PCO_2 ratio. Similarly, a change in PCO_2 caused by a respiratory disorder will alter the [HCO_3]. In most of the acid-base disturbances chemical buffering alone is not sufficient to restore normal pH. Respiratory and renal compensation will then restore to near normal pH. The lung can respond within minutes by increasing or decreasing ventilation but renal compensation takes hours or days. In acute respiratory disorders, which affect CO_2 concentration pH change is considerable. If the disorders are chronic renal compensation occurs by reabsorption and regeneration of new bicarbonate and PH will return to near normal. Arterial blood gas measurement allows us,

1. To interpret the oxygenation status (PO_2) and
2. The acid-base status (pH, PCO_2) of a patient.

    Interpretation of acid-base enables us to make deductions about the derangements in respiratory function.

Oxygenation Status

In health the partial pressure of oxygen in arterial blood (PaO_2) is close to the partial pressure of oxygen in the pulmonary alveoli (PaO_2). In disease processes affecting the respiratory system, PaO_2 can be very different from PaO_2.

ASSESSMENT OF ACID BASE DISORDER (FIG. 16.1)

Identification of an acid-base disorder is to understand the severity of the underlying pathophysiologic mechanisms and guide treatment.

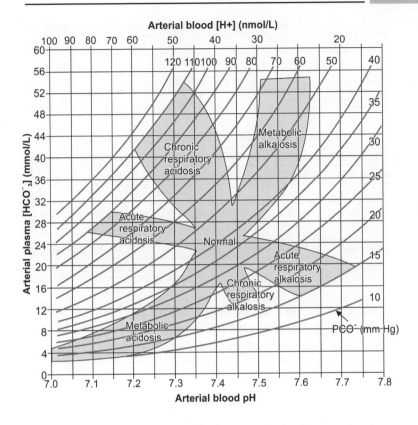

Fig. 16.1: Acid-Base nomogram indicating approximate reference values for common disturbances

- Acidosis and alkalosis are processes, that cause derangements in H^+ ion concentration, acidemia and alkalemia respectively in the steady-state acid base status of the body. Various respiratory and metabolic disorders cause changes in hydrogen ion concentration, $[H^+]$.
- $[H^+]$ is commonly expressed as pH, which is the negative logarithm of $[H^+]$.
- $[H^+]$ in body fluids is extremely low - measurable in nanomoles per liter (Table 16.1).
- Respiratory disorders change pH by causing primary changes in PCO_2 and metabolic disorders alter acid concentrations or $[H^+$ ions].

Table 16.1: Normal acid-base values

Parameter	Range	Optimal value
pH	7.35–7.45	7.40
PCO_2 (mm Hg)	36–44	40
Bicarbonate (millimoles/L)	22–26	24

Table 16.2: Range of H⁺ ions in plasma in clinical conditions

	pH	H⁺nmol/L	Remarks
Range	7.35–7.45	35–45	normal
Optimal value	7.40	40	
Acidemia	7.1–7.3	50–80	Clinically important
Acidemia	< 7	> 100	Can be fatal
Alkalemia	7.46–7.69	20–36	Clinically important
Alkalemia	> 7.7	< 20	Can be fatal

Range of H⁺ ions in plasma in clinical conditions is shown in Table 16.2. Primary changes in PCO_2 are responsible for respiratory acidosis or respiratory alkalosis. Primary changes in HCO_3 or changes in acid concentration can cause metabolic acidosis or metabolic alkalosis.

An acid-base disorder occurs with

a. Change in respiratory or renal function or

b. Addition of acid or alkali to extracellular fluid.

The most common method of interpretation of acid-base dysfunction is based on Henderson-Hasselbalch equation. This is by analyzing the HCO_3/PCO_2 ratio. The four primary abnormalities can exist either singly or in combination with each other (Mixed acid-base disorder).

(The term 'non-respiratory' is used instead of 'metabolic' to denote that we cannot deduce a metabolic disorder from considering pH and PCO_2 alone.)

In primary respiratory acid-base disorders, pH and PCO_2 are inversely proportional. In respiratory acidosis, pH is decreased and PCO_2 is increased. In respiratory alkalosis, pH is increased but PCO_2 is decreased. In metabolic abnormalities, pH and

Table 16.3: pH, PCO_2 and acid-base status

pH	PCO_2	Acid-Base status
Normal	Normal	Normal
Increased	Increased	Non-respiratory alkalosis
Increased	Decreased	Respiratory alkalosis
Decreased	Increased	Respiratory acidosis
Decreased	Decreased	Non-respiratory acidosis

HCO_3 change in the same direction. Loss of HCO_3 or addition of an acid result in metabolic acidosis whereas addition of HCO_3 or loss of acid results in metabolic alkalosis (Table 16.3). CO_2 transport profoundly affects the acid-base status of blood. The lungs excrete about 10,000 mmol of carbonic acid as CO_2 daily compared with 20–70 mmol/day of non-volatile acid excretion by the kidneys. Therefore, if ventilation is stopped suddenly, respiratory acidosis can develop in minutes but the metabolic acidosis of acute renal failure takes hours or days to develop. CO_2 partial pressure is controlled by chemoreceptors in the medulla controlling the rate and depth of breathing. In metabolic acidosis when pH decreases, the CSF acidity will also decrease and this will stimulate the chemoreceptors of medulla. The rate and depth of respiration will increase and will try to minimize changes in pH by reducing PCO_2. This occurs immediately within minutes and hence the compensation is complete. On the other hand in a respiratory disorder renal compensation takes time. When respiratory disturbances occur acutely, the compensation is not complete where as in chronic respiratory disorders the metabolic compensation is complete. This respiratory response to change in pH occurs acutely, normally within minutes. Renal compensation for a primary respiratory disorder takes longer and it is therefore possible to distinguish between acute and chronic respiratory disorders, depending on whether renal compensation has occurred or not. There are different methods for analyzing the respiratory and metabolic components of acid-base disorders.

1. Boston Approach—the CO_2-HCO_3 ('Boston') Approach

This uses the relationship between PCO_2 and HCO_3 as defined by the Henderson-Hasselbalch equation.

2. Winter's Formula

The expected HCO_3 for any given pH and PCO_2 in respiratory disorders and expected PCO_2 for any given pH and HCO_3 can be calculated using winter's formula:

$PCO_2 = [(HCO_3 \times 1.5) + 8] \pm 2$

This approach gives accurate results in simple respiratory and metabolic acid-base disorders and indicates the presence of a mixed disorder when the actual value of PCO_2 or HCO_3 falls outside the expected range.

Anticipated changes in PCO_2 and HCO_3 for changes in HCO_3 and PCO_2 follow some rule and is shown below:

Respiratory compensation for a metabolic disorder and renal compensation for a respiratory disorder have been observed clinically to follow some rules as tabled below:

The expected values can be found out for any given change in PCO_2 and HCO_3 using the above nomogram. In simple acid-base disorders, the measured value will be the same as expected value. A deviation of the measured value from the expected value indicates a mixed acid-base disorder. A triple acid-base disorder is diagnosed when metabolic acidosis and alkalosis co-exists with either respiratory acidosis or respiratory alkalosis.

3. The Base Deficit/Excess ('Copenhagen') Approach

Base excess or base deficit is used to identify the type of acid-base disorder. In respiratory disorder the base excess (BE) is normal (within ± 2 mmol/L). In metabolic disorder the base excess is outside the above value.

4. Buffer-Base (1948, Singer and Hastings)

Buffer-base (1948, Singer and Hastings) is the sum of the nonvolatile weak anions plus bicarbonate. It is similar in concept to the modern strong ion difference.

5. Standard Bicarbonate (1960, Astrup)

Standard Bicarbonate (1960, Astrup) is the bicarbonate which is standardized for a PCO_2 of 40 mm Hg. This is calculated using the Henderson-Hasselbalch equation. The measured pH and PCO_2 of 40 mm Hg is substituted in the above equation to calculate *Standard bicarbonate.*

6. Base Excess (1960, Siggaard-Andersen and Engel)

Base excess (1960, Siggaard-Andersen and Engel) was defined as the amount of titrable acid required to bring the pH to 7.4 at a PCO_2 of 40 mm Hg.

The Siggaard-Andersen nomogram derived from studies in volunteers and the Van Slyke equation to calculate base excess are incorporated into blood gas analyzers.

The *anion gap* concept was devised to differentiate between different types of metabolic acidosis.

Anion gap is $([Na^+] + [K^+]) - ([Cl-] + HCO_3^-])$ and is normally positive (8 to 16 mEq/L) because there is less unmeasured anion than unmeasured cation.

The normal anion gap is contributed by unmeasured anions such as phosphate and protein. The gap is widened (high anion gap metabolic acidosis) when there is an accumulation of excess anions such as ketone bodies in DKA or lactate in sepsis. Anion gap will be normal if acidosis is due to a low bicarbonate and high chloride as in renal tubular acidosis.

7. The Stewart-Fencl Approach

The Stewart-Fencl approach analyses acid-base from principles of physical chemistry and is an attractive concept. It is very accurate than other available methods. Unfortunately, its application involves polynomial algebraic equations and requires a computer. This approach is discussed later in another chapter.

The *anion gap approach* complements the other approaches. Calculation of the anion gap should be a routine part of the examination for every set of electrolytes.

The anion gap is equal to the difference between the plasma concentrations of the major cation sodium (Na) and the major measured anions chloride and bicarbonate ($Cl^- + HCO_3^-$).

The normal value of the anion gap is approximately 12 ± 2.

The usual unmeasured anion consists of albumin, and therefore the normal anion gap changes in the setting of hypoalbuminemia. Normal anion gap is approximately three times the serum albumin in g/dL.

Because the total number of cations must equal the total number of anions, a fall in the serum HCO_3^- concentration must be offset by a rise in the concentration of other anions. If the anion accompanying excess H^+ is Cl^- then the fall in the serum HCO_3^- concentration is matched by an equal rise in the serum Cl^- concentration. The acidosis is classified as a normal gap or hyperchloremic metabolic acidosis. By contrast, if excess H^+ is accompanied by an anion other than Cl^-, then the fall in HCO_3^- is balanced by a rise in the concentration of the unmeasured anion. The Cl^- concentration remains the same. In this setting, the acidosis is said to be a high anion gap metabolic acidosis. An increase in the anion gap can occur whenever there is an increase in unmeasured anions (increased valency of albumin, hyperphosphatemia) or a decrease in the unmeasured cations (hypocalcemia, hypomagnesemia). However, the most common cause of an increase in anion gap is the generation of a metabolic acidosis by addition of a non-Cl acid. It uses the difference between anions and cations of the commonly measured electrolytes Na^+, K^+, Cl^- and HCO_3^-:

$$(Na^+ + K^+) - (Cl^- + HCO_3^-)$$

This anion gap exists because unmeasured anions amounting to 8–16 mEq/L exist in normal conditions. If the gap widens to > 16 then there is an excess of unmeasured anion. AG has to be adjusted for serum albumin concentration otherwise high AG metabolic acidosis will be missed. A correction formula for low serum albumin is

Anion gap (corrected) = anion gap + 2.5 (normal albumin – patient's albumin in g/dL)

Calculations of both base deficit and anion gap can underestimate or miss an alkalosis caused by hyperventilation because they rely on bicarbonate values and bicarbonate is lowered by a low PCO_2.

The *delta anion gap* ratio is calculated in the presence of a high anion gap metabolic acidosis to identify a mixed disorder. The delta anion gap is the difference between observed AG and normal AG. This is compared to delta HCO_3 which is the difference between normal HCO_3 and observed HCO_3. If delta AG is more than delta HCO_3 it suggest metabolic alkalosis. Delta HCO_3 more than delta AG is diagnostic of hybrid metabolic acidosis (combination of non AG metabolic acidosis and AGMA).

The delta gap (or ratio) is the difference (or ratio) between the patient's anion gap and bicarbonate (HCO_3)

Delta ratio = Δ Anion gap/Δ [HCO_3^-] = (anion gap – 12) ÷ (24-HCO_3) (assuming normal AG = 12, Normal HCO_3 = 24)

One molecule of unmeasured acid is added to ECF it dissociates and the extra H^+ ions added combines with HCO_3 which gets converted to H_2O + CO_2. So for each 1 mmol of acid added, 1 mmol of HCO_3 is reduced by buffering. However, in vivo, about 50% of buffering takes place intracellularly so change in anion gap is not equal to the change in HCO_3. In diabetic ketoacidosis, acid is lost in the urine and the delta ratio is close to one.

In lactic acidosis the ratio is about 1.6.

A delta ratio < 1 indicates the decrease in HCO_3 is greater than the increase in anion gap - **occurs when anion gap acidosis coexist with non anion gap acidosis.**

A delta ratio > 2 indicates a preexisting elevated HCO_3, so a coexisting metabolic alkalosis or compensated respiratory acidosis is likely.

INTERPRETATION OF ARTERIAL BLOOD GAS (ABG)

A practical assessment of a patient's acid-base status involves the following steps:

1. Clinical assessment will include a detailed history physical examination and preliminary investigations.
2. pH < 7.35: It is academia, > 7.45: It is alkalemia. pH can be normal in mixed acid-base disorder.
3. The primary change is either in PCO_2 or HCO_3. The change in the other parameter is the compensatory response. The change in pH corresponds to the primary change.

   Acidosis — high PCO_2 or low HCO_3

   Alkalosis — low PCO_2 or high HCO_3

   The compensatory response must be in the same direction as the initial change, i.e. for a high PCO_2, the HCO_3 increases in compensation. *If the response is in the opposite direction there is a mixed disorder.* Calculate the degree of compensation according to standard rules as shown in Table 16.4.
4. In metabolic acidosis calculate anion gap and if elevated calculate delta ratio to look for a mixed disorder.
5. Formulate a unified diagnosis based on clinical assessment, initial investigations, acid-base changes and confirmatory investigations.

   Measurements of body fluid chemistry made from blood or plasma are indicative of their concentrations in ECF since plasma and ECF are freely miscible for small molecules. ICF concentrations are very different and controlled by membrane channels and pumps (Table 16.5).

Table 16.4: Initial changes and compensations in simple acid-base disorders

Disorder	HCO$_3$	PCO$_2$	Compensation
Metabolic acidosis	Primary decrease	Compensatory decrease	Winter's formula PCO$_2$ = [(HCO$_3$ × 1.5) + 8] ± 2
Metabolic alkalosis	Primary increase	Compensatory increase	0.7 mm Hg rise in PCO$_2$ for each 1 mmol/L rise in HCO$_3$
Respiratory acidosis	Compensatory increase	Primary increase	Acute: 1 mmol/L rise in HCO$_3$ for each 10 mm Hg rise in PCO$_2$ Chronic: 3.5 mmol/L rise in HCO$_3$ for each 10 mm Hg rise in PCO$_2$
Respiratory alkalosis	Compensatory decrease	Primary decrease	Acute: 2 mmo/L fall in HCO$_3$ for each 10 mm Hg fall in PCO$_2$ Chronic: 4 mmol/L fall in HCO$_3$ for each 10 mm Hg fall in PCO$_2$

Table 16.5: Extracellular fluid composition (ECF) in mEq/L

Cations	mEq/L	Anions	mEq/L
Na	142	Cl	101
K	4	HCO$_3$	27
Ca	5	PO$_4$	3
Mg	2	Protein	16
H	0.004	Organic acid	6

Intracellular fluid composition (ICF) in mEq/L

Cations	mEq/L	Anions	mEq/L
Na	10	Cl	3
K	160	HCO$_3$	10
Ca	2	PO$_4$	100
Mg	26	SO$_4$	20

ECF and ICF composition (adapted from http://cats.med. uvm.edu/physiology/body fluids)

DEFINITIONS

Acid: Bronsted and Lowry's definition. An acid is a substance that donates a proton and base is a substance that accepts a proton in a reaction.

pH— pH is a measure of the acidity or basicity of an aqueous solution.

The term pH was suggested by Sorensen (1909).

Defined as the negative logarith am$_{10}$ of the H$^+$ ions concentration expressed in gram ions per liter.

pH = – log [H$^+$]

Pure water is said to be neutral, with a pH close to 7.0 at 25°C (77°F). Solutions with a pH less than 7 are said to be acidic and solutions with a pH greater than 7 are basic or alkaline.

Acidosis: Describes the processes by which H$^+$ ions are added to system or alkali is removed but because of effective buffering, hydrogen ion concentration does not increase or decrease and pH will be normal.

Acidemia: When hydrogen ion concentration increase above 45 nmoles and the pH falls below 7.35, condition is termed acidemia.

Alkalosis: Describes the process by which alkali is added or H$^+$ ions are removed from the system but because of effective buffering hydrogen ion concentration does not decrease or and there is no change in pH.

Alkalemia: When hydrogen ion concentration decrease below 35 nmoles and when the pH increases above 7.45, condition is Alkalemia.

Acidosis-acidemia, Alkalosis-alkalemia are used interchangably.

Buffers: Buffer confers resistance to changes in the pH of a solution when hydrogen ions (protons) or hydroxide ions are added or removed. An acid-base buffer typically consists of a weak acid, and its conjugate base (salt). For a buffer system to be effective the concentration should be large when compared to the amount of protons or hydroxide ions added or removed. This optimal buffering occurs when the pH is within approximately 1 pH unit from the pK value for the buffering system, i.e. when the pH is between 5.1 and 7.1.

HENDERSON EQUATION (DESCRIBED IN 1908)

Henderson's equation quantitates the relationship between $[H^+]$, $[HCO_3^-]$, and PCO_2

$$[H^+] [HCO_3^-] = K \times PCO_2$$

$$[H^+] = \frac{K \times PCO_2}{[HCO_3^-]}$$

Henderson Hasselbalch Equation (described in 1916) gives the derivation of pH as a measure of acidity using pKa, the acid dissociation constant

Hasselbalch used pH for H^+ions in Henderson's equation form

$$pH = pKa + \frac{Log\ ([A^-])}{([HA])}$$

Applying to bicarbonate carbonic acid buffer system,

The Henderson-Hasselbalch equation can be written as

$pH = pKa + log\ HCO_3/PCO_2$

The Henderson-Hasselbalch equation indicates that pH depends on the ratio of HCO_3^-/PCO_2. pH increases when the ratio increases (alkalosis), and pH decreases when the ratio decreases (acidosis). The ratio may be increased by an increase in HCO_3^- (metabolic alkalosis) or by a decrease in PCO_2 (respiratory alkalosis).

The ratio may be decreased by a decrease in HCO_3^- (metabolic acidosis) or by an increase in PCO_2 (respiratory acidosis).

Bicarbonate in ABG report- ABG analyzer measures pH and pCO_2. Bicarbonate is calculated using modified Henderson's Equation.

$[H+] = 24 \times [pCO_2]/[HCO_3^-]$,

hence $[HCO_3^-] = 24\ [pCO_2]/[H^+]$,

At the normal $[H^+]$of 40 nmol/L and pCO_2 of 40 mm Hg, by applying modified Henderson's Equation,

$HCO_3^-] = 24 \times 40/40 = 24$ nmoles/L

Example: If H^+ions = 30 and pCO_2= 60 mm Hg, HCO_3 can be calculated using the equation,

$HCO_3 =, HCO_3 = 24 \times 60/30 = 48$

Some times ABG measurements (pH, pCO_2) may be wrong. To check the accuracy of these measurements, H^+ ions can be calculated from Henderson's equation using the measured bicarbonate, (bicarbonate can be measured directly and this value can be inserted in the Henderson's equations). The calculated value of H^+ ions and the measured H^+ ion should be identical if the ABG measurement is accurate. Measured bicarbonate is within 2–4 millimoles of calculated value of bicarbonate by the analyzer, the report is correct.

In the above example, the measured bicarbonate was 40 and calculated using Henderson's equation was 48, this indicates that ABG measurement is not correct.

Interconversion of H^+ Ions and pH

Since the ABG analyzer gives pH, this has to be converted into H ions. Few conversion tables are shown below. Hydrogen ion concentration and corresponding pH values.

$[H^+]$ mol/L	pH
79×10^{-9}	7.10
71×10^{-9}	7.15
63×10^{-9}	7.20
56×10^{-9}	7.25
50×10^{-9}	7.30
45×10^{-9}	7.35
40×10^{-9}	7.40
35×10^{-9}	7.45
32×10^{-9}	7.50
28×10^{-9}	7.55

pH varies inversely with hydrogen ion concentration. Within the physiological pH range of 7.35 to 7.45 the $[H^+]$ changes only a little from 45 to 35 nmol/L but with a pH of 7.2 which is commonly seen clinically, the $[H^+]$ has risen to more than 1½ times. [H⁺] thus can be seen to rise steeply with acidosis.

Other Formulae to Convert H⁺ Ions into pH

Rule of Thumb 1

Between pH 7.28 and 7.55 there is a linear relationship between pH and H⁺ ions.

Drop 7 and decimal point, find out the difference between 40 and the number. If pH is < 7.4, add the difference to 40 and if pH is > 7.4, subtract the difference from 40.

Example 1: To convert 7.28 into H ions,
Step 1: Drop 7 and decimal, number is 28.
Step 2: Find out the difference between 40 and 28, 40–28 = 12
Step 3: As pH decreases, H ions increase as they are inversely proportional. Add 12 to 40 (normal H ion concentration)
40 + 12 = 52 pH 7.28 corresponds to H⁺ ion concentration of 52 nmoles/L
Example 2: To convert 7.55 into H ions,
Step 1: Drop 7 and decimal, number is 55
Step 2: Find out the difference between 40 and 55, 55–40 = 15
Step 3: As pH increases, H ions decrease as they are inversely proportional. Subtract 15 from 40 (normal H ion concentration) 40–15 = 25. pH 7.55 corresponds to H⁺ ion concentration of 25 nmoles/L

pH values and corresponding hydrogen ion concentration Conversion based on rule of thumb 1

pH	[H⁺] nmol/L
7.28	52
7.29	51
7.3	50
7.35	45
7.4	40
7.45	35
7.5	30
7.51	29
7.52	28
7.55	25

Rule of Thumb 2—the 0.1 Change in pH Rule.

For every 0.1 increase in pH above 7.0 multiply by 0.8 and decrease in pH by 0.1 multiply by 1.25.

pH of 7 = 100 nmol/L

> **Example 1:** If pH is 7.1, H ions = 100 × 0.8 = 80 nmol/L,
> **Example 2:** pH 7.2 = 100 × 0.8 × 0.8 = 64
> **Example 3:** pH 6.9 = 100 × 1.25 = 125

pH	H ions nmol/L
7	100
6.9	100 × 1.25 = 125
6.8	100 × 1.25 × 1.25 = 156
6.95	Between 100 and 125, 112
7.1	100 × 0.8 = 80
7.2	100 × 0.8 × 0.8 = 64
7. 15	Between 80 and 64, 72

Normal blood gas values		
pH	Arterial pH	7.40
$PaCO_2$	Arterial pCO_2	40 mm Hg
PaO_2	Arterial pO_2	98 mm to 100 Hg
HCO_3^-	Arterial bicarbonate	24 ± 2 mmol/L
	Venous bicarbonate	28 ± 2 mmol/L

Importance of pH in clinical conditions			
Condition	pH	H^+ ions in nmol/L	Importance
Acidemia	< 7	100	Can be lethal - urgent
Acidemia	< 7.2	< 64	Requires treatment
Normal	7.4 ± 0.0 2	40 ± 2	Normal
Alkalemia	7.44	– 7.69	20–36 Requires treatment
Alkalemia	> 7.7	< 20	Can be lethal - urgent

KEY POINTS

- There are four primary acid-base abnormalities.
- Compensatory (secondary) processes restore pH toward normal in response to one or more primary acid-base abnormalities; the kidneys compensate for primary respiratory disorders, and the lungs compensate for primary metabolic disorders.
- A *simple* acid-base disorder is caused by a single *primary* abnormality with appropriate physiologic compensation.
- *Mixed* acid-base disorders result from multiple primary processes. Up to 3 of the 4 primary processes can coexist, but respiratory acidosis and respiratory alkalosis are mutually exclusive.
- Metabolic acidosis is further classified into normal AG and elevated AG varieties.

The Stewart Approach to Acid-Base

G Krishnakumar

Because pH is easily measured and HCO_3 is printed on the blood gas report we tend to think of these values as 'primary'. The Henderson-Hasselbalch equation also gives us the impression that pH (and therefore acid-base status) is determined solely by the ratio of HCO_3 to PCO_2. However, other variables such as serum proteins, phosphate, sulfate and many others also affect the hydrogen ion concentration ($[H^+]$). The traditional approach to analysis of acid-base balance is descriptive rather than analytical and could possibly miss some complex mixed disorders.

Based on physicochemical principles, Stewart determined the acid-base status in detail of different concentrations of various mixtures of solutes. According to these studies, the hydrogen ion concentration ($[H^+]$) of blood is determined by the strong ion difference (SID), PCO_2, and total weak acid (A_{tot}). These are independent variables and they affect the concentrations of dependent variables such as HCO_3 and OH. Thus it was shown that $[H^+]$ is not determined by bicarbonate concentration but vice versa. Respiratory disorders affect $[H^+]$ by changes in PCO_2 and metabolic disorders by changes in SID and A_{tot}.

Pure water has a neutral pH of 7 at 25°C and a slightly lower pH of 6.8 at 37°C. This change of pH of pure water with change in temperature occurs because temperature affects the dissociation of water molecules into H^+ and OH^-.

A solution of HCl and NaOH in water has Na, Cl, H and OH ions. Na⁺ and Cl⁻ being 'strong ions' dissociate completely in solution. Such a mixture will not have equal quantities of Na and Cl ions if the molar amounts of HCl and NaOH are not equal. For such a solution Stewart's equations show that [H⁺] (and therefore pH) is determined by the difference between Na⁺ and Cl⁻ concentrations.

$$[H^+] = [Na^+] - [Cl^-]$$

Weak acids such as phosphate and negatively charged proteins do not dissociate completely in solution and exist as both dissociated (A⁻) and undissociated (HA) forms. For more complex solutions containing weak anions in addition to strong cations like K⁺, Mg⁺⁺, Ca⁺⁺ and strong anions like Cl⁻ and lactate (in physiological solutions lactate is considered a strong ion), the pH is determined by the difference between the sum of the strong cations and the strong anions. This value is called the strong ion difference:

$$SID = [Na + K + Mg + Ca] - [Cl + lactate]$$

This can be represented graphically (Fig. 17.1):

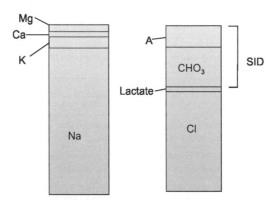

Fig. 17.1: Graphical representation of ions in normal plasma: The vertical bars indicate cations and anions and are equal in height because plasma is electrically neutral. PCO2 affects pH but is depicted here in only its ionic form, HCO3. H⁺ and OH − are not shown because their concentrations are in nanomoles, too small to be seen on the bars. Lactate concentration is also very small in normal conditions but is shown because it is significant in illness.

Stewart derived a complex polynomial equation to express $[H^+]$ in terms of the independent variables: $[H^+]^4 + [H^+]^3\{Ka + [SID]\} + [H^+]^2\{Ka\,([SID]\,[A_{tot}]) - (K_C \times PCO_2 + K_W)\}\,[H^+]\{Ka(K_C \times PCO_2 + K_W) + K_3 \times K_C \times PCO_2\}\,Ka \times K_3 \times K_C \times PCO_2 = 0$.

(Where Ka, K_3, K_C, and K_W are dissociation constants for A_{tot}, carbonate, bicarbonate and water respectively).

Figge and Fencl have derived an even more complex equation to describe the dissociation properties of different amino acid residues on the albumin molecule and citrate. These equations are too difficult to calculate manually and require an iterative computer program to solve them. However, it is possible to understand the principles involved without much mathematics.

The Table 17.1 lists commonly used terms of acid-base physiology.

Table 17.1: Definitions and abbreviations (modified from Rastegar, Clin J Am Soc Nephrol 4: 1 267 – 1274, 2009)

AG = anion gap = $([Na^+]+[K^+]) - ([Cl^-]+[HCO_3])$ (normal range 14–16) or AG = $([Na^+] - ([Cl^-]+[HCO_3])$ (normal range 8–12)
AG_c = AG corrected for albumin = observed AG + $(2.5 \times \{4.4 -$ observed albumin in g/dL})
A^- = anions mostly phosphate + albumin in plasma (also haemoglobin in whole blood)
A_{tot} = total A^- and its weak acids $[A^-] + [HA]$
Buffer-base = $([Na^+]+[K^+]+Ca^{2+} + Mg^{2+}) - ([Cl^-] = [HCO_3+A^-]$
Base excess/deficit = BE/BD = amount of acid/alkali that must be added to 1 liter blood to restore pH to 7.4 at 37° C and PCO_2 of 40 mm Hg
Standard BE/BD = BE/BD corrected for Hb and size of interstitial fluid compartment. Calculated as actual BE/BD ÷ 3 or with Hb 5 g/dL
SID = strong ion difference = $([Na^+]+[K^+]+ Ca^{2+}+ Mg^{2+}) - ([Cl^-]$ = $[HCO_3+A^-]$ SID_a = apparent SID = $([Na^+] + [K^+]+ Ca^{2+}+ Mg^{2+}) - ([Cl^-]$)
SID_e = effective SID = $[HCO_3+A^-]$ = $[HCO_3]$ + $(0.2\,8 \times$ albumin g/L) + (1.8 × phosphate mmol/L)
SIG = strong ion gap = SID_a ." SID_e

The major practical difference between Stewart's approach and the traditional approach is the use of SID and SIG to understand metabolic disorders, rather than bicarbonate and anion gap.

When an abnormal anion is present (Fig. 17.2) a difference exists between SID calculated as $([Na^+]+[K^+]+Ca^{2+}+Mg^{2+}- [Cl^-])$ (apparent SID) and SID calculated as the sum of (bicarbonate + albumin + phosphate) (effective SID). The difference between SID_a and SID_e is the strong ion gap, SIG — more appropriately called net unmeasured anions. SIG is very close to anion gap corrected for albumin. Ideally, if there are no unmeasured ions SID_a and SID_e should be equal and SIG should be zero.

In the presence of complex mixed disorders, especially alkalosis due to hypoalbuminemia the calculation of SIG may reveal the presence of metabolic acidosis even with a normal bicarbonate and BE. Hypoalbuminemia and metabolic acidosis are both common in the critically ill and the former can mask the latter.

It can be seen from the diagram above that a change in SID can change A^- and HCO_3, with or without a change in SIG which is something we commonly observe — for example a anion gap metabolic acidosis such as diabetic ketoacidosis (high SIG, low bicarbonate).

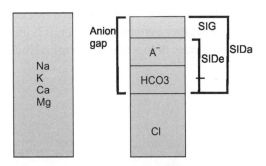

Fig. 17.2: Graphical representation of ions in metabolic acidosis
Anion gap is albumin + phosphate + other unmeasured anions = (A^-) + other unmeasured anions if present (>16 mmol/L). SIG is numerically very close to anion gap corrected for albumin and phosphate. It represents net unmeasured anions other than A^-.

Table 17.2: Changes in SID, A_{tot}, and PCO_2 in primary acid-base disturbances

Parameter	Acidosis	Alkalosis
Respiratory	$\uparrow PCO_2$	$\downarrow PCO_2$
Non-respiratory: Altered SID		
Water excess/deficit	$\downarrow$ SID $\downarrow$ Na	$\uparrow$ SID $\uparrow$ Na
Chloride excess/deficit	$\uparrow$ Cl $\downarrow$ SID	$\downarrow$ Cl $\uparrow$ SID
Unmeasured anions	$\uparrow$ unmeasured	$\downarrow$ unmeasured anion
	anion $\downarrow$ SID	$\uparrow$ SID
Non-respiratory: Altered A_{tot}		
Albumin	$\uparrow$ albumin	$\downarrow$ albumin
Inorganic phosphate	$\uparrow$ P	$\downarrow$ P

In respiratory disorders, change in [H$^+$] is due solely to change in PCO_2 but in metabolic disorders [H$^+$] can change as a result of changes in SID or A_{tot} (see Table 17.2).

Thus, the Stewart approach can be seen to explain the mechanisms of some phenomena which are not well understood using the traditional approach, for example:

Hyperchloremic acidosis: Increase in Cl$^-$ decreases SID
Hypoproteinemic alkalosis: Decrease in A$^-$ increases HCO$_3$, Cl being unchanged.

There have been several studies comparing patients treated on the basis of analysis of data with Stewart's approach with that of control groups and these have not convincingly demonstrated a mortality benefit. However, it is an interesting alternative point of view of this complex topic which is gaining many supporters.

Metabolic Acidosis

A Vimala

OVERVIEW

Normal arterial pH is 7.35 – 7.45. The intracellular fluid (ICF) pH is between 7.0 and 7.3. Intracellular fluid (ICF) is more acidic than ECF. Normal acid production is 1 mEq/kg. Most important buffer in ECF is bicarbonate buffer system and in ICF is protein buffer system. Early morning urine pH is around 5.4 and normal anion gap is 12 mmol ± 2 mmol/L. Metabolic acidosis can be the only acid-base abnormality, i.e., simple acid base disorder or can coexist with other abnormalities as mixed acid-base disorder. Most common associated abnormality is respiratory alkalosis. Metabolic acidosis can be classified into anion gap metabolic acidosis and non-anion gap metabolic acidosis (hypercholremic metabolic acidosis). Correction of acidosis should be very judicious and pH < 7.1 need only be corrected. Overcorrection can produce cardiac arrhythmias, and carry high mortality.

DEFINITION AND MECHANISM

This is a process where there is an over production of H^+ ions and resultant decrease in bicarbonate due to buffering. Hydrogen ions can be produced either endogenously or by exogenous addition of acids or precursors of acids like alcohols. Primary abnormality in metabolic acidosis is decrease in bicarbonate concentration. Bicarbonate concentration can decrease by loss of bicarbonate or increase in ECF volume.

Decrease of Bicarbonate

1. *Reduction in bicarbonate due to buffering of H^+ ions:* Endogenous over production of organic acids as in diabetic keto-acidosis or exogenous addition of acids as in methyl alcohol poisoning can result in addition of excess H^+ ions to ECF. These H^+ ions will be buffered by bicarbonate. Bicarbonate concentration will decrease.

2. *Primary decrease in bicarbonate:* Gastrointestinal loss of bicarbonate in stools as in diarrhea or decreased reabsorption of bicarbonate by the renal tubules can result in low bicarbonate.

3. *Dilution of bicarbonate:* In fluid overload states, when ECF volume expands the normal bicarbonate content gets diluted in larger volume of ECF and bicarbonate concentration will be low.

Consumption of Organic Acids, Alcohol or Endogenous Production of Excess of Organic Acids

When an organic acid is added exogenously or endogenously H^+ ions are added. With the addition of 1 molecule of organic acid, it combines with HCO_3 to form carbonic acid. Carbonic acid will dissociate into carbon dioxide and water. The organic anion is excreted in urine. CO_2 is eliminated by lungs. Hence, approximately 1 molecule decrease in HCO_3 will result in decrease in 1 molecule of PCO_2.

$$\text{organic acid} + HCO_3 \Rightarrow H_2CO_3 + \text{organic anion}$$
$$\Downarrow$$
$$H_2O + CO_2.$$

Reduction of HCO_3 in Plasma due to Loss through GI Tract or Kidney

When 1 molecule of bicarbonate is lost through gastro intestinal tract as in diarrhea, or due to decreased reabsorption of bicarbonate by the renal tubules, 1 molecule of chloride is reabsorbed to maintain electroneutrality. So when bicarbonate is lost, 1 chloride molecule is gained. Hence, sum of anions will remain constant.

Addition of Non-bicarbonate Solutes

Non-bicarbonate solutes are added to ECF, the ECF volume expands. Bicarbonate get diluted in a larger volume of ECF and concentration of bicarbonate decreases and this results in expansion acidosis.

Expected PCO$_2$ in Metabolic Acidosis

Rule of Thumb 1

For every 1 molecule reduction in HCO$_3$ from 24, PCO$_2$ also will decrease by 1 mm of Hg.

Example: If HCO$_3$ decreases from 24 to 18 mmol/L.PCO$_2$ also will decrease by 6 mm Hg. Expected PCO$_2$ is 34 mm Hg.

Rule of Thumb 2

From the pH, value drop the number 7, the last 2 numbers will be the expected PCO$_2$.

Example: If pH is 7.40, the expected PCO$_2$ is 40 mm Hg. If pH is 7.32, the expected PCO$_2$ is 32 mm Hg.

Rule of Thumb 3

Expected PCO$_2$ = [(HCO$_3$ × 1.5) + 8 ±] 2.
HCO$_3$ is 24, PCO$_2$ = [(24 × 1.5) + 8 ±] 2 = 44 ± 2

Rule of Thumb 4

Add 15 to HCO$_3$ value to get the expected PCO$_2$.

PCO$_2$ = 24 + 15 = 39 mm Hg
If HCO$_3$ is 20, expected PCO$_2$ is 35 mm Hg.

If the expected PCO$_2$ as per the nomograms and the measured PCO$_2$ are different, a mixed acid-base disturbance is present. If the measured PCO$_2$ is less than expected PCO$_2$, it indicates hyperventilation and washing out of CO_2. The abnormality is respiratory alkalosis. If the measured PCO_2 is more than expected PCO_2, it indicates hypoventilation and accumulation of CO_2. The abnormality is respiratory acidosis.

ANION GAP (AG) IN METABOLIC ACIDOSIS

What is Anion Gap? (Fig. 18.1)

Anion gap (AG) is the difference between measured cations and measured anions. Anion gap is based on the principle of electroneutrality which states that in any solution.

Sum of concentration of Cations = Sum of concentration of anions

Plasma contains both cations and anions and the sum of cations should always be equal to sum of anions to maintain electroneutrality.

In plasma cations that are usually measured are Na^+, K^+, Ca^+, Mg^+ and anions that are usually measured are Cl^- and HCO_3^-. There are other unmeasured cations and anions. Hence, equation can be written as Anion gap (AG).

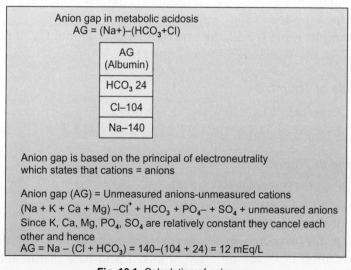

Fig. 18.1: Calculation of anion gap

$AG = \{Na^+ + K^+ + Ca^+ + Mg^+\}$ + Unmeasured cations –
$\{Cl^- + HCO_3^- + PO_4^- + SO_4^-\}$ + unmeasured anions

Since K, Ca, Mg, PO_4, SO_4^- are relatively small in concentration and constant, they cancel each other.

Na^+ + unmeasured cations = Cl^- + HCO_3^- + unmeasured anions
Unmeasured anions -Unmeasured cations

= Na^+ – (Cl^- + HCO_3^-)
Hence AG = (Na^+) – (HCO_3^- + Cl^-)

{Na^+ is sodium concentration, HCO_3^- is bicarbonate concentration, and Cl^- is chloride concentration; all concentrations are in mmol/L}

Normal AG = 140 – (24 + 104) = 12 mmol/L

If potassium is also taken in the calculation,

Normal AG = (140 + 4) – (24 + 104) = 16 mmol/L

The anion that is not included in the calculation is albumin and AG is **mainly due to albumin**. AG changes with changes in Albumin concentration.

High Anion Gap Metabolic Acidosis (AGMA) (Fig. 18.2)

This is due to addition of organic acids. As discussed earlier, when excess of organic acids are added,

$HA \rightarrow H^+ + A^-$. The added H ion will combine with HCO_3 and form carbonic acid.

This is unstable and will dissociate into CO_2 and H_2O. Thus, 1 molecule of organic acid will result in decrease of 1 molecule

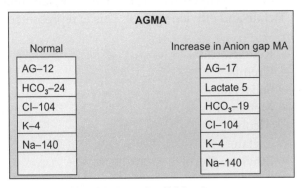

AGMA	
Normal	Increase in Anion gap MA
AG–12	AG–17
HCO_3–24	Lactate 5
Cl–104	HCO_3–19
K–4	Cl–104
Na–140	K–4
	Na–140

Fig. 18.2: Example of high anion gap

of bicarbonate and increase of 1 molecule of unmeasured anion. The organic anion cannot enter the cell and hence is excreted by the kidney.

Example: When 5 molecules of lactic acid are added to plasma, **5 (H^+ lactate$^-$) ⇨ 5 H^+ + 5 lactate$^-$)** These H^+ ions are buffered by bicarbonate buffer system.

$$5\ H^+ + 5\ HCO_3 ⇨ 5\ H_2CO_3 ⇨ 5\ H_2O + 5\ CO_2$$

and HCO_3 will decrease from 24 to 19 mmol/L. $\Delta\ HCO_3$ is the difference between normal HCO_3 and observed HCO_3.

So in the above example, **Delta HCO_3 = 24 – 19 = 5**

Anion gap = $Na^+ - [Cl^- + HCO_3^-]$

AG = {140 – 104 + 19 +} = 17

The anion gap is 17 and is due to lactate molecules that are added but not usually measured.

Δ **AG is the difference between observed anion gap and normal anion gap. In this example, Δ AG = 17 – 12 = 5.**

$\Delta\ HCO_3 = \Delta\ AG = 5$

In Anion gap metabolic acidosis, $\Delta HCO_3 = \Delta$ AG

If K is included,

AG = ($[Na^+]$ + $[K^+]$) – ($[Cl^-]$ – $[HCO_3^-]$)

Causes of increase in AG is shown in Figure 18.3.

AG = unmeasured anions – unmeasured cations, hence increase in anion gap can be due to an increase in unmeasured anions or decrease in unmeasured cations.

Common causes for increase in unmeasured anions are

Ketoacidosis (DM, starvation), uremia, salicylate, methanol, alcohol, lactate and ethylene glycol. This is represented by the acronym.

K – Ketoacidosis
U – Uremia
S – Salicylate
M – Methanol
A – Alcohol
L – Lactate
E – Ethylene glycol

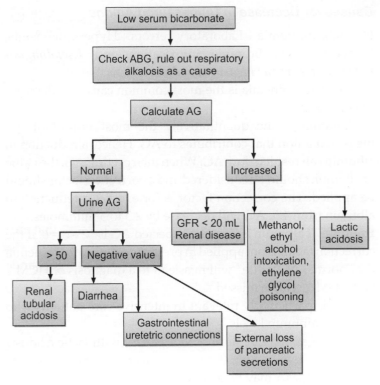

Fig. 18.3: Assessment of low HCO_3 concentration

Common causes for decrease in unmeasured cations are Hypocalcemia, hypomagnesemia, hypokalemia
Metabolic alkalosis: In metabolic alkalosis AG can increase by 2 to 3. This is due to change in charge of protein.

Causes of Decrease in Anion Gap

Causes of decrease in anion gap are increase in unmeasured cations or decrease in unmeasured anions.

Causes for Increase in Unmeasured Cations

Hyperkalemia, hypercalcemia, hypermagnesemia, lithium intoxication, and high IgG levels.

Causes for Decrease in Unmeasured Anions

Hypoalbuminemia, Laboratory errors, Hyperproleinemia, Hyperlipidemia, Bromide intoxication and *Pseudohyponatremia where the measured sodium is low.*

Hypoalbuminemia is the most common cause for decrease in anion gap

Albumin is the quantitatively the most important unmeasured anion that contributes to AG. Hence, a reduction in albumin can result in low AG. When interpreting AG, the value of albumin should be considered and a correction factor should be applied. The correction factor is for every 1 g reduction in albumin from 4.5, AG will decrease by 2.5 to 3 millimoles.

Example: If albumin is 2.5 g the expected AG is 12 – 6 = 6. If the correction factor is not applied in presence of hypoalbuminemia the "normal AG value" will misslead to a diagnosis of HCMA and AGMA will be missed.

This is particularly relevant in intensive care patients who have low albumin levels.

Anion gap may be normal in a patient with lactic acidosis if Albumin level is low. If correction factor is not applied for albumin, AGMA may be missed.

Case History 1

A 50-year-old patient with diabetic nephropathy is admitted with fever and dyspnea.

Date	On Admission
Urineprotein	+ +
Hb, TC	13.9, 14200 (N93L$_7$)
RBS	550 mg/dL
Urea	121 mg/dL
Creatinine	2.6 mg/dL
Na	131 mmol/L
K	4 mmol/L
Cl	96 mmol/L
Alb	4.4 g/L

ABG parameters	On the day of admission
pH	7.24
PCO_2	28 mm Hg
paO_2	86% on room air
BE	–5.7
BE ecf	–28.5
HCO_3	12.0 mmol/L
O_2sat	92%

What is the ABG disorder?

The following steps are used for evaluating the ABG abnormality

1. Interpret the pH – pH is 7.24, is lower than normal, hence has acidosis.
2. Correlate the change in the pH with change in HCO_3^- pH is low and HCO_3 is low, hence has metabolic acidosis
3. Expected PCO_2 for the change in bicarbonate is 28 (for every mmol decrease in HCO_3, PCO_2 decreases by 1 mm. Here the expected PCO_2 and measured PCO_2 are the same, hence diagnosis is *simple metabolic acidosis.*
4. Calculate the anion gap, AG = 131 – (96 +12), = 23 AG is increased, Hence metabolic acidosis is classified as (AGMA).

Diabetic Ketoacidosis (DKA)

This is a consequence of uncontrolled hyperglycemia and is seen in 8 to 29% of hospitalized diabetic patients.

Clinical Presentation

Patients are usually dehydrated. They present in a stuporous state and breath has a fruity odor. Respiration is rapid and sighing which is described as Kussmaul's respiration.

An important non-surgical cause for acute abdomen is diabetic keto acidosis.

Precipitating Factors are: Infection, non-compliance to insulin therapy and diet, cardiovascular events, pancreatitis or cocaine abuse.

Differential diagnosis of DKA include:

- Hyperosmolar non-ketotic diabetes
- Lactic acidosis
- Uremic acidosis

Laboratory abnormalities commonly seen are shown below:

Parameters	Variable
Glucose	> 250 mg/dL Exceptions are pregnancy malnutrition and alcoholism
HCO_3	< 15 mmol/L
S Na	Decreased (1.6 mmol decrease for every 100 mg increase in glucose above 100
S. K	Low or normal (total body K decreased)
pH	< 7.35
CO_2	< 30 mm Hg
AG	> 10

Treatment

- Hyperglycemia induces osmotic diuresis. Patients are dehydrated due to loss of water and electrolytes. Estimated total fluid deficit is 100 mL/kg body weight. Mainstay of treatment is correction of fluid deficit. Rapid infusion of one liter of normal saline over 1 hour can be given.
- Total fluid given should not exceed $4L/m^2/24$ h
- Correction of hyperglycemia is with intravenous insulin infusion. It is started at the rate of 3 units/h and dose is adjusted by frequent monitoring of glucose levels in blood.

OSMOLAL GAP

Osmolal gap is the difference between measured plasma osmolality and calculated osmolality.

Plasma osmolality is contributed by osmotically active solutes in plasma. Osmotically active solutes in plasma are glucose, urea, sodium and potassium.

The formula for calculation of osmolality is

$$\frac{\text{Glucose in mg/dL}}{18} + \frac{\text{urea in mg/dL}}{6} + 2\,[\text{Na} + \text{K}]$$

Osmolality is dependent on the number of osmotically active particles. To find out the number of osmotically active particles concentrations in mg/dL has to be converted into millimoles. Molecular formula of glucose is $C_6H_{12}O_6$ and molecular weight is 180. 180 g of glucose dissolved in 1 liter of water is 1 mole of glucose. 18 mg dissolved in 100 mL is 1 mmol.

Molecular formula of urea is $NH_2\text{-CO-}NH_2$ and hence molecular weight is 60. If 60 g of urea is dissolved in 1 liter of water this is 1 mole of urea. That is 6 mg dissolved in 100 mL is 1 mmol.

Sodium chloride and potassium chloride will dissociate in to Na, K and Cl respectively. Each molecule of NaCl and KCl will dissociate into two osmotically active particles. Hence concentration of Na and K are multiplied by 2.

The accurate way of determining osmolality is by measuring plasma osmolality using osmometer.

Osmolal gap = measured osmolality – calculated osmolality. Normally the osmolal gap is around 10. If the osmolal gap is more than 10, suspect the presence of osmotically active particles like methyl alcohol, ethylene glycol, etc. The toxin does not produce an increase in osmolal gap is toluene.

Metabolic Acidosis Caused by Toxins

Methanol Intoxication

Methyl alcohol is a common cause of intoxication.
Methyl alcohol gets oxidized to formaldehyde and formic acid.

$$CH_3OH \xrightarrow{\text{Hepatic dehydrogenase}} HCHO \rightarrow HCOOH$$

Principles in the treatment of methanol intoxication include:
1. Decreasing the metabolism of methyl alcohol to its toxic metabolite formaldehyde

2. Correction of acidosis and
3. Removal of methanol

1. Decreasing the Metabolism of Methyl Alcohol to its Toxic Metabolite Formaldehyde

- Ethyl alcohol is used as a therapeutic agent to arrest the metabolism of methanol. Ethyl alcohol (ethanol) has hundred times more affinity for hepatic alcohol dehydrogenanse than methyl alcohol. Therapeutic level of ethanol in blood has to be maintained for the duration of intoxication.

Dose of Ethyl alcohol
- In chronic drinkers 0.15 g/kg/hr intravenously or 60 mL of whiskey/h orally.
- In non-drinkers 0.07 g/kg/h intravenously or 30 mL of whiskey/h orally.

Desired therapeutic level of ethanol is 22 mmol/L.

2. Correction of Acidosis

Acidosis is corrected with sodium bicarbonate if arterial pH is < 7.

3. Removal of Alcohol

Hemodialysis is indicated for removal of methyl alcohol if level of methyl alcohol is more than 50 mg/L.

NON-ANION GAP METABOLIC ACIDOSIS (HYPERCHLOREMIC METABOLIC ACIDOSIS)

This is associated with a normal anion gap, a decrease in plasma bicarbonate concentration, and an increase in plasma chloride concentration. As discussed earlier, when there is
- increased loss of bicarbonate in stools as in diarrhea
- or defective reabsorption of bicarbonate and or impaired secretion of H^+ ions as in renal tubular acidosis there will be a corresponding increase in chloride reabsorption.

Case History 2

A 10-year-old student is admitted with diarrhea and dyspnea. ABG revealed

Date	On Admission
Urine protein	nil
Hb, TC	13.9, 7500
RBS	102 mg%
Urea	60 mg%
Creatinine	0.9 mg%
Na	130 mmol/L
K	2.6 mmol/L
Cl	117 mmol/L
Alb	4.4 g/L

ABG parameters	On the day of admission
PH	7.16
PCO_2	23
PO_2	96 mm on room air
BE	–5.7
BE ecf	–28.5
HCO_3	8.0 mmol/L
O_2sat	98%

What is the ABG disorder?

The following steps are used for evaluating the ABG abnormality

1. Interpret the pH – pH is 7.16, is very low, hence acidosis
2. Correlate the change in the pH with change in HCO_3^- pH is low and HCO_3 is low (8 millimoles), hence has metabolic acidosis
3. Expected PCO_2 for the change in bicarbonate is 24 (for every mmol decrease in HCO_3, PCO_2 decreases by 1 mm.) Here the expected PCO_2 and measured PCO_2 are the same, hence diagnosis is *simple metabolic acidosis*
4. Calculate the anion gap, AG = 130 – (8 +117), = 5 AG is normal suggesting Non-Anion-Gap metabolic acidosis – Hyperchloremic metabolic acidosis

Approach to Hyperchloremic Metabolic Acidosis

Hyperchloremic metabolic acidosis can result from loss of bicarbonate through GI tract, defective bicarbonate reabsorption and or H^+ ion secretion by renal tubules. To find out the route of loss of bicarbonate, urine anion gap (urine AG) is calculated.

Urine Anion Gap (Urine AG) - Urine Net Charge

What is Urine AG? (Fig. 18.4)

As in plasma, urine also contains positive charges and negative charges and to maintain electroneutrality, sum of concentration of cations should be equal to sum of concentration of anions

The cations normally present in urine are Na^+, K^+, NH_4^+, Ca^{++} and Mg^{++}.

The anions normally present are Cl^-, sulfate, phosphate and some organic anions. *Bicarbonate is not present in normal urine.* The usually measured cations are sodium and potassium and anion that is measured is chloride. The cation that is quantitatively significant in urine but not measured usually is ammonium NH_4^+, NH_4 is excreted as NH_4 Cl.

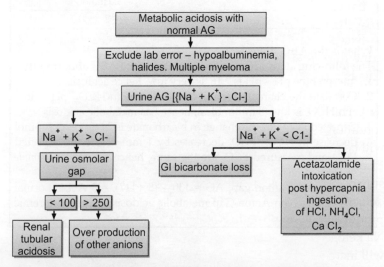

Fig. 18.4: Approach to metabolic acidosis with normal anion gap

The cation NH_4 is not normally measured, but the accompanying anion Cl^- is measured.

Based on the principle of electroneutrality, total anion charge always equals total cation charge.

Hence equation can be written as

$Na^+ + K^+$ + unmeasured cation (UC) = Cl^- + unmeasured anions (UA)

Since Na and K are the most abundant cations and chloride abundant anion, equation can be rearranged as

Urinary Anion Gap = $[Na^+] + [K^+] - [Cl^-]$.

In extra renal **HCMA,** the kidneys are functioning normally, the excess H^+ ions are lost in urine as ammonium to maintain normal pH. If NH_4 excretion in urine is plentiful, and this will be excreted as NH_4 Cl and measured Cl^- will be much greater than the sum of Na^+ and K^+. The negative anion gap will indicate excretion of NH_4 in urine.

In renal causes of HCMA, kidneys will not respond appropriately by excreting H^+ ions in urine as NH_4. The sum of Na^+ and K^+ concentration will be greater than chloride. So to summarize,

$[Cl^-] > [Na^+] + [K^+]$ = High NH_4 in urine

$[Cl^-] < [Na^+] + [K^+]$ = low NH_4 in urine or excretion of NH_4 with an anion other than Cl^-.

Exceptions: When unusual anions are to be excreted in urine this will lead to increase in sodium excretion in urine. This is because the anions are excreted as sodium salts. Here the accompanying anion is not measured, hence $[Cl^-] < [Na^+] + [K^+]$. This does not indicate *impaired ammonia excretion*. In such conditions the differentiation is easy because the anion gap will be increased.

Example: Diabetic ketoacidosis is a clinical situation where the sum of excretion of Na^+ and K^+ is $>Cl^-$ but this does not indicate defective NH_4 excretion. This is because when ketoacids are produced in excess and lost in urine, ketoacetate is excreted as Na ketoacetate. If 10 molecules of ketoacids are lost urine, Na^+ will increase by 10.

This will lead to an increase in urine anion gap but this can easily by diagnosed by measuring plasma anion gap which will also be increased.

Clinical Application of Urine Anion Gap (Fig. 18.4)

Non-AG metabolic acidosis (**hyperchloremic metabolic acidosis**) can result from either renal or extra renal cause.

The urinary anion gap helps to differentiate between GIT and renal causes of HCMA.

Normal response of kidneys to metabolic acidosis is to excrete excess H⁺ ions as NH₄.

Net acid excretion is the difference between bicarbonate loss and bicarbonate gain. Bicarbonate loss is found out from urinary NH_4 and HPO_4 excretion.

Net acid excretion (NAE) =
Bicarbonate loss – bicarbonate gain = $NH_4^+ + H_2PO_4 - HCO_3$

In extra renal causes of acidosis urinary NH_4 excretion will increase. Urine will contain more NH_4 which is excreted as NH_4 Cl and can increase to 300 to 400 milli Moles. In urine the accompanying anion chloride which is measured will also increase to the same extent. So [Cl⁻] will be greater than the sum of [Na⁺] + [K⁺] and urine AG is negative.

A negative value of urine AG suggests increased renal NH₄ excretion and is suggestive of extra renal causes for acidosis.

In non-anion gap acidosis due to renal disease, the renal compensation does not occur and NH_4 excretion in urine will not increase. The cations Na⁺, K⁺ excretion will increase

Hence **[Cl⁻] < [Na⁺] + [K⁺] = low ,NH₄ in urine**

A positive value of urine AG suggests decreased renal NH₄ excretion and is suggestive of renal causes for acidosis.

Osmolar Gap in Urine

Urine osmolality is mainly contributed by urea, sodium and potassium.

$$\textbf{Urine osmolality} = \frac{\text{Urea in mg/dl}}{6} + 2\,[Na + K]$$

If urine contains 1500 mg of urea, 50 mmoles of Na and 50 moles of K,

$$\text{Urine osmolality} = \frac{1500\ \text{mg/dl}}{6} + 2\,[\,50 + 50\,] = 250 + 200$$

$$= 450\ \text{millimoles}$$

Accurate estimation of osmolality is by measuring osmolality using osmometer. This is based on the principle of freezing point depression. Osmolal gap is the difference between measured osmolality and calculated osmolality.

Osmolal gap = [Measured osmolality-calculated osmolality]

In conditions like Diabetic keto acidosis, large number of anions are excreted in urine. Since these anions are not usually measured, these are not taken into consideration, while calculating urine osmolality. When osmolality is measured using osmometer, urine osmolality will be very high. If the measured osmolality is 800 milliosmoles and calculated osmolality is 450, the osmolar gap is 350. Urine NH_4 excretion can be found out by multiplying osmolar gap by 0.5, since 50% of the osmolal gap is contributed by NH_4 in urine.

Case History 3

A 65-year-old patient with history of diabetes mellites developed fever, rigor and abdominal pain, He was treated with antibiotics following which he developed diarrhea.

Laboratory parameters in blood are shows below

Na	132 mmol/L
K	2.8 mmol/L
Cl	115 mmol/L
HCO_3	11 mmol/L
Albumin	4 gms/L
AG	132 – [115 + 11] = 6
pH	7.24
pCO_2	26

Contd...

	Contd...
PO$_2$	96 mm on room air
HCO$_3$	11 mmol/L
O$_2$sat	98%

What is the ABG disorder?

The following steps are used for evaluating the ABG abnormality

1. Interpret the pH – pH is 7.24, is very low, hence patient has aciodosis
2. Correlate the change in the pH with change in HCO$_3^-$ pH is low and HCO$_3$ is low (11 mmol/L) hence has metabolic acidosis
3. Expected PCO$_2$ for the change in bicarbonate is 26 (for every mmol decrease in HCO$_3$, PCO$_2$ decreases by 1 mm). Here the expected PCO$_2$ and measured PCO$_2$ are the same, hence diagnosis is *simple metabolic acidosis*
4. Calculate the anion gap, AG = 132 – (11 + 115), = 6 AG is normal suggesting non-anion gap metabolic acidosis (Hyperchloremic metabolic acidosis).

   In this patient, acidosis can be due to tubulionterstitial nephritis or diarrhea.
5. Find out urine anion gap (AG)

Urine Electrolytes	
Na+	15
K$^+$	50
Cl$^-$	100
Urine AG - (Na$^+$ + K$^+$) - Cl	–35

Urine AG is negative. Suggest normal renal response. So the probable cause for acidosis in this patient is diarrhea.

MANAGEMENT

Indication for Alkali Treatment

In acidosis associated with chronic kidney disease aim is to maintain plasma bicarbonate concentration within 20 to 22 mmol/L.

Correction of Acute Metabolic Acidosis

Decision to treat acute metabolic acidosis is decided by the severity of acidosis and rapidity of development. Goal is to keep the pH between 7.1 and 7.15. Sodium bicarbonate either oral or parenteral is used for correction of metabolic acidosis. Dose of sodium bicarbonate required depends on the volume of distribution of HCO_3. Volume of distribution will vary depending on the arterial pH. Between 7.3 to 7.4, distribution space is 50% of the lean body weight (LBW). If the pH is less than 7.1 volume of distribution is 100% of the body weight.

Available Preparations

Intravenous preparation: 1 mL contains 0.9 millimoles.
10 mL = 9 mmoles
This is also available as 8.5% solution.
10 mL will contain = 10 mmoles

Calculation of the Deficit

Bicarbonate deficit can be calculated as follows
- Dose of bicarbonate required = (24 – patient's bicarbonate) × 100% of LBW in severe acidosis. 50% of the requirement has to be given in the first 24 hours.
- Bicarbonate can be given intravenously as bolus in hypertonic states. In patients, who are volume depleted 150 mmoles of $NaHCO_3$ has to be added to 1 liter of 5% dextrose solution. This will make it an isotonic solution.

KEY POINTS

- Metabolic acidosis is due to primary decrease in bicarbonate concentration.
- This can be classified into AGMA and Non-AG metabolic acidosis (HCMA).
- Serum albumin should always be considered in the interpretation of AG.
- Non-AG metabolic acidosis can be further classified based on urine AG.
- Positive urine AG value indicates renal cause and negative value indicates non-renal cause.
- Presence of osmolal gap in urine indicate presence of usually unmeasured anions.
- Acute correction of acidosis is indicated only if pH is < 7.15. ·

CHAPTER 19

Metabolic Alkalosis

R Kasi Visweswaran, A Vimala

OVERVIEW

This is a common but under recognized problem encountered in hospitalized patients. This accounts for approximately 50% of all acid-base disorders. Severe metabolic alkalosis (i.e. blood pH > 7.55) is associated with a mortality of 45 to 80%. pH > 7.65 is lethal.

Metabolic alkalosis can be classified into saline responsive and saline non-responsive alkalosis. The most common cause of metabolic alkalosis is ECF volume contraction – 'Contraction alkalosis'. As discussed earlier, normal renal and pulmonary function play a key role in maintaining the bicarbonate level in the blood within the narrow range of 24–26 mEq/L. We will briefly discuss the classification, pathophysiology, and an algorithmic approach to arrive at etiology and management.

DEFINITION

Metabolic alkalemiais is manifested as increase in arterial pH more than 7.45 due to primary increase in plasma bicarbonate (HCO_3^-) concentration. This may or may not be associated with compensatory increase in $PaCO_2$. Metabolic alkalosis is the term used to describe the process in which the bicarbonate is in excess but is buffered, so that the pH is maintained in the normal range. This can be understood from the Henderson-Hasselbalch equation

pH = PKa + log HCO_3/$PaCO_2$ and Henderson's equation

H^+ ions = 24 × $PaCO_2$/HCO_3. In metabolic alkalosis, primary change is increase in HCO_3 which is the denominator of the Henderson's equation. To keep H^+ ions constant, numerator $PaCO_2$ will have to increase (same direction rule). This is by the compensatory adaptive mechanism of hypoventilation and thereby increasing $PaCO_2$. This occurs immediately. Thus, pH is maintained below 7.45. The respiratory adaptive mechanism is followed by renal adaptive mechanism. Excess of bicarbonate will be excreted with conservation of Cl⁻ ion. Thus, metabolic alkalosis is transient and gets corrected in a short time. When the buffering mechanism is inadequate, pH increases above normal range > 7.45. This condition is termed alkalemia. *Alkalosis and alkalemia are used interchangeably.* In this chapter, alkalosis is used for alkalemia also.

Metabolic alkalosis can occur as a single abnormality or as a component of other acid-base abnormalities metabolic acidosis, respiratory acidosis or respiratory alkalosis.

Expected $PaCO_2$ for a given Increase in Bicarbonate

Arterial $PaCO_2$ increases by 0.7–0.75 mm Hg for every one mEq/L increase in plasma bicarbonate concentration, a compensatory response that is very quick.

Simple formula for finding out expected $PaCO_2$ for a given increase in bicarbonate

Expected $PaCO_2$ between the concentrations of HCO_3 from 10–40 mmol/L can be calculated using the simple formula

$$PaCO_2 = HCO_3 + 15$$

1. If HCO_3 is 40, the expected $PaCO_2$ = 55
2. If HCO_3 is 34, the expected $PaCO_2$ = 49
3. If HCO_3 is 25, the expected $PaCO_2$ = 40 (normal)
4. If HCO_3 is 14, the expected $PaCO_2$ = 29
5. If HCO_3 is 10, the expected $PaCO_2$ = 25.

ABG analyzer measures directly only pH and $PaCO_2$. HCO_3 is calculated using Henderson's equation $HCO_3 = 24 \times PaCO_2/H^+ions$. Bicarbonte can also be measured in venous blood.

Measured total carbon dioxide content in venous blood is higher than the calculated bicarbonate in arterial blood by 1-3 mEq/L. This is because tissue metabolism generates bicarbonate. In addition it also measures dissolved PCO_2. Thus, at a $PaCO_2$ of 40 mm Hg, the contribution by dissolved PCO_2 alone will be $(0.03 \times 40) = 1.2$ mm Hg.

Does high bicarbonate always indicate metabolic alkalosis?

No, bicarbonate can also increase as a compensation to respiratory acidosis. This can be differentiated by measuring arterial pH. To find out whether the increase in HCO_3 is due to metabolic alkalosis or compensation to respiratory acidosis— Correlate with arterial pH. pH > 7.45 and raised bicarbonate suggest metabolic alkalosis, pH < 7.35 and raised bicarbonate suggest respiratory acidosis.

WHY TO RECOGNIZE METABOLIC ALKALOSIS?

Unrecognized and untreated metabolic alkalosis leads to serious clinical sequelae resulting in increased morbidity and mortality. Sequelae are

Cerebral insufficiency due to hypoxia: There are two mechanisms by which hypoxia is caused.

- Alkalosis shifts the oxygen saturation curve to the left thereby impairing oxygen delivery to the tissues resulting in tissue hypoxia. Alkalosis causes depression of the respiratory center. This is a physiologic response to alkalosis to retain CO_2 and thus to keep pH within normal limits. Depression of the respiratory center can also exacerbate this hypoxia.

Hypocalcemia

Calcium exists in ionized form and bound form. Ionized calcium is the physiologically active form of calcium. The bound form depends on albumin concentration. Alkalosis increases the binding of calcium to protein anions and reduce the fraction of ionized calcium. This can trigger headache, lethargy, and sometimes patient may present with delirium, neuromuscular excitability, tetany and seizures.

Hypomagnesemia

Alkalosis can also be associated with hypomagnesemia. It should be suspected in patients who present with seizures refractory to calcium infusions and may respond only to parenteral magnesium.

Angina

Alkalosis produces vasoconstriction. This vasoconstrictive effect on the diseased coronary artery results in exacerbation of angina.

Cardiac Arrhythmias

The electrolyte abnormalities associated with metabolic alkalosis can precipitate cardiac arrhythmias. There is increased risk for *cardiac arrhythmias in patients with sepsis syndrome on renal replacement therapy*. The usual abnormality in a patient with sepsis syndrome and acute kidney injury is metabolic acidosis and respiratory alkalosis. Hemodialysis will sometimes over correct metabolic acidosis to metabolic alkalosis. If the already existing respiratory alkalosis due to sepsis is not recognized and corrected, patients can develop combination of metabolic alkalosis and respiratory alkalosis driving the pH further away from normal leading to catastrophic consequences and result in profound hypokalemia, hypocalcemia, hypomagnesemia, and sudden cardiac arrest.

Muscle Weakness

Hypokalemia may cause muscle weakness.

CLASSIFICATION AND APPROACH

Metabolic alkalosis can be classified based on GFR and ECF volume. Metabolic alkalosis usually develops in patients with normal GFR and rare in patients with decreased GFR. Normal response to decrease in GFR is metabolic acidosis (Fig. 19.1).

Metabolic alkalosis can occur in decreased GFR when associated with

- Injudicious alkali ingestion, infusions, incessant vomiting
- Sodium polystyrene sulfonates used along with aluminium hydroxide (Fig. 19.1).

Pathogenesis of Metabolic Alkalosis

Two processes are involved in the development of metabolic alkalosis. *Either loss of non-volatile acid from ECF or gain of alkali.* It is not common for alkali to be added to the body.

The disorder involves a generative stage—whereby alkalosis is generated by loss of acid and a maintenance stage in which the kidneys fail to excrete bicarbonate.

Generation of Metabolic Alkalosis

This occurs usually when there is loss of non-volatile acid and reduction in ECF volume.

Pathogenesis of alkalosis in ECF volume contraction: There are two mechanisms by which metabolic alkalosis is generated.

1. Contraction of extracellular fluid volume results in redistribution of bicarbonate in a smaller volume of fluid,

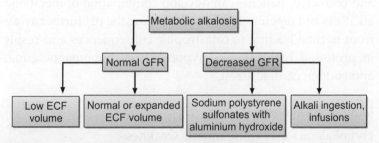

Fig. 19.1: Causes based on GFR

and an increase in bicarbonate concentration. This causes, at most, a 2 to 4 mEq/L rise in bicarbonate concentration. Metabolic alkalosis can be corrected by expanding ECF volume with saline infusions. Acid infusions are not indicated.

2. The second mechanism is failure of kidneys to excrete excess bicarbonate. When ECF volume contracts, the normal physiological response is retention of Na^+ ions by the kidney. When sodium has to be reabsorbed an anion has to accompany. In chloride depletion, the accompanying anion is bicarbonate, with resultant increase in bicarbonate concentration. This leads to generation of metabolic alkalosis.

Case History 1

A 60-year-old lady admitted with history of chronic obstructive pulmonary disease (COPD) and pneumonia, has the following ABG values.

pH	7.31
$PaCO_2$	55 mm Hg
HCO_3	26 mmol/L
PaO_2	70 mm Hg

Stepwise Approach

1. pH is decreased–normal range is (7.35–7.45) indicating increase in H^+ ions, hence acidemia.
2. HCO_3 is 26 which is above the normal range of 22–24 mmol/L -indicates retention of bicarbonate
3. Is it due to metabolic alkalosis?

To find out whether the increase in HCO_3 is due to metabolic alkalosis or compensation to respiratory acidosis — Correlate with arterial pH. Here the bicarbonate is high, $PaCO_2$ high and pH is low < 7.35. This indicates the primary abnormality is retention of CO_2 from hypoventilation and bicarbonate retention is secondary to renal response to minimize the change in pH due to respiratory acidosis.

Case History 2

A 3-month-old child weighing 4 kg is admitted with vomiting. On examination the child was hypovolemic, blood pressure in the 95th percentile and ECF deficit was assessed to be around 100 mL.

Investigations are as follows

Parameters in blood/serum	Values
Blood urea	28 mg%
Creatinine	0.6 mg%
Na	120 mmol L
K	3 mmol L
Chloride	94 mmol/L
Bicarbonate	32 mmol/L

Child has hyponatremia, hypokalemia, hypochloremia and raised bicarbonate

The next step is to obtain ABG

pH	7.45
PCO_2	47 mm Hg
HCO_3	32 mmol/L
PaO_2	96 mm Hg

Stepwise Approach

Step 1: Interpret the pH. pH is 7.45, indicating decrease in H^+ ions hence alkalosis.

Step 2: Correlate pH with HCO_3^-. pH is high, bicarbonate is also high indicating metabolic alkalosis.

Step 3: What is his $PaCO_2$? 47 mm Hg (above normal, value of 40 mm Hg). To recapitulate, arterial $PaCO_2$ increases by 0.7–0.75 mm Hg for every 1 mEq/L increase in plasma bicarbonate concentration. In this child, plasma HCO_3 is 32 mmol/L, expected increasein $PaCO_2$ is $(32 - 24) \times 0.7$–$0.75 = 5.6$ to 6 mm Hg (applying simple formula, $32 + 15 = 47$). So the expected $PaCO_2$ is $40 + 5.6 = 45.6$ to 47 mm Hg. Expected $PaCO_2$ and obtained $PaCO_2$ are almost identical, indicating that the pulmonary response is appropriate and hence this is a simple acid-base disorder—Simple metabolic alkalosis

What is the cause of metabolic alkalosis? *Can this high bicarbonate concentration be due to ECF volume contrction alone?*
Normal total bicarbonate in ECF = 0.933 × 24 = 22.4 mmol.
Now 22.4 mmol of bicarbonate is redistributed in 833 mL of ECF instead of 933 mL, new bicarbonate concentration is 22.4/00.833 liters × 1 L = 26.9 mmole/L (Fig. 19.2).

If increase in bicarbonate was only due to volume contraction alone, bicarbonate concentration should have been 26.9. Obtained bicarbonate concentration is 32 mmol/L, hence increase in bicarbonate is not due to redistribution of bicarbonate in a smaller volume of fluid alone.

Step 3: To find out whether ECF volume contraction is causing alkalosis, estimate urine chloride concentration. Urine chloride < 25 mEq/L, suggests renal mechanism is intact and probable cause of alkalosis is extrarenal

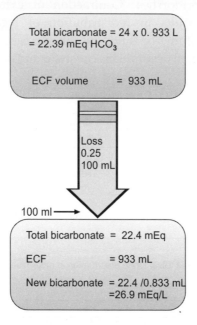

Total bicarbonate = 24 x 0. 933 L
= 22.39 mEq HCO_3

ECF volume   = 933 mL

Loss
0.25
100 mL

100 ml ⟶

Total bicarbonate = 22.4 mEq

ECF   = 933 mL

New bicarbonate = 22.4 /0.833 mL
=26.9 mEq/L

Fig. 19.2: Increase in HCO_3 with decrease in ECF volume case history 2

Total body water in the child = body weight × 0.7 = 4 × 0.7= 2.8 Liters. Normal ECF volume = 1/3rd of total body water = 2.8 × 1/3rd = 933 mL. After loosing 100 mL, current ECF volume = 933 − 100 = 833 mL

Classification of causes based on urine chloride concentration is shown in Table 19.1.

Urine electrolytes of this child (case history 2) is shown in Table 19.2.

Urine chloride is **8 mmol/L**. This child with hypochloremia is conserving chloride and the route of loss is extrarenal.

The probable cause is vomiting from gastric outlet obstruction, pyloric stenosis.

Contraction Alkalosis

1. Metabolic alkalosis due to ECF volume contraction can be due to loss of extracellular fluid rich in chloride and poor in bicarbonate. Common causes are vomiting, diuretic therapy (thiazides, loop diuretics) and rarely from chloridorrhea. Contraction of extracellular fluid volume results in redistribution of bicarbonate in a smaller volume of fluid, and an increase in bicarbonate concentration occurs. This causes, at most, a 2 to 4 mEq/L

Table 19.1: Causes based on urine chloride loss

Less than 25 mEq/L	Greater than 40 mEq/L
Vomiting/nasogastric suction	Primary mineralocorticoids
Diuretics (late)	Diuretics (early)
Factitious diarrhea	Alkali load (HCO_3^-/other organic anion)
Posthypercapnia Cystic fibrosis Low chloride intake	Bartter's /Gitelman's syndrome severe hypokalemia (2 mEq/L)

Table 19.2: Urine electrolytes in case history 2

Electolytes in urine	mMoles/L
Na+	15
K+	30
Cl-	8

rise in bicarbonate concentration. Metabolic alkalosis can be corrected by expanding ECF volume with saline infusions. Acid infusions are not indicated.

2. Loss of hydrogen ions: Whenever, a hydrogen ion is excreted, one bicarbonate ion is gained into the extracellular space.

Hydrogen ions may be lost through the kidneys or the GI tract. Vomiting or nasogastric (NG) suction generates metabolic alkalosis by the loss of gastric secretions, which are rich in hydrochloric acid (HCl).

The physiological response of kidney, when bicarbonate level increases is to increase the excretion of bicarbonate. Mechanisms involved are:

1. Increase in bicarbonate (HCO_3) is associated with volume expansion, which reduces reabsorption of sodium ions and bicarbonate ions in the proximal tubule and bicarbonate is brought back to normal.

2. Stimulation of bicarbonate secretion by the chloride/HCO_3 exchanger: The kidneys secrete the excess bicarbonate via the apical chloride/bicarbonate exchanger in the β-type intercalated cells of the collecting duct. Protons are gained to the systemic circulation via the basolateral H^+ATPase.

Metabolic alkalosis develops when the physiological mechanisms fail and kidneys are unable to excrete excess bicarbonate.

Factors that reduce bicarbonate excretion are:

ECF Volume Contraction (Fig. 19.3)

1. Leads to reduction in GFR and reduction in filtered load of HCO_3

2. Activation of RAAS— Angiotensin 11 stimulates reabsorption of bicarbonate

3. Stimulation of sympathetic nervous system.

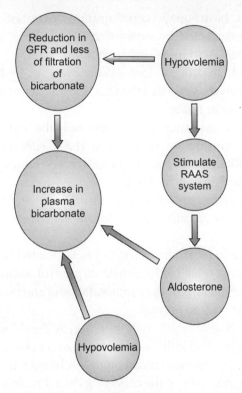

Fig. 19.3: Mechanism of ECF volume contraction induced increase in bicarbonate

Maintenance of Metabolic Alkalosis

Once the metabolic alkalosis is generated, this will be maintained if the following conditions exist. Factors playing a role are hypovolemia, chloride depletion, hypokalemia and renal loss of hydrogen ions.

Hypovolemia

Besides the factors mentioned above hypovolemia also prevents loss of bicarbonate in urine by increased activity of the apical proton pump through aldosterone. Whenever a hydrogen ion is secreted into the tubular lumen, a bicarbonate ion is gained into the systemic circulation via the basolateral Cl/HCO_3 exchanger.

Chloride Depletion

This will stimulate the renin angiotens aldosterone system. In the late thick ascending limb and early distal tubule, specialized cells are present. These cells have $Na^+/K^+/2Cl$ cotransporters in the apical membrane. This is mainly regulated by chloride ions. In chloride depletion states, the macula densa (modified myoepithelial cells of the afferent arteriole) secrete renin. This increases aldosterone secretion via angiotensin II leading to reabsorbtion of bicarbonate.

Renal Loss of Hydrogen Ions

When the distal delivery of sodium increases increased aldosterone stimulates the electrogenic epithelial sodium channel (ENaC) in the collecting duct. As this channel reabsorbs sodium ions, the tubular lumen becomes more negative, leading to the secretion of hydrogen ions and potassium ions into the lumen.

Hypokalemia

- Increases H^+ion secretion in the distal nephron and decreases bicarbonate loss.
- Stimulates ammonia production which enhances renal excretion of hydrogen ions by the proximal tubule.

GENERATION AND MAINTENANCE OF METABOLIC ALKALOSIS IN SPECIFIC SITUATIONS

Vomiting and Nasogastric Suction

Loss of gastric juice can result in metabolic alkalosis. Around 1500 mL of gastric juice is secreted in 24 hours. Gastric juice contains more chloride than sodium.

Composition of Gastric Juice

Volume	1200 mL/24 h
Na	60 mmol/L
K	10 mmol/L
Cl	130 mmol/L

Gastric juice does not contain bicarbonate

In normal **basal state**, volume of gastric juice secreted is 50 mL/h. (approximately 1200 mL in 24 hours) H_2CO_3 formed from CO_2 and H_2O, dissociates into H^+ ions and HCO_3^-. H^+ is secreted into gastric juice and HCO_3^- is retained in ECF. The HCO_3^- retained in ECF is lost in pancreatic juice and intestinal secretions there by maintaining the balance of H^+ ions in the body.

In conditions like pyloric stenosis around 1–2 liters of gastric juice is lost through vomitus resulting in loss of H^+ ions. The factors maintaining metabolic alkalosis are:

1. ECF Volume Contraction

In vomiting, Na, Cl and water are lost leading to ECF volume contraction. Since more chloride is lost in gastric juice than Na, the amount of chloride filtered is less. This leads to a reduction in Cl⁻ in luminal fluid. Na reabsorption occurs, the anion that accompanies is HCO_3 and plasma HCO_3 concentration increases. This maintains metabolic alkalosis. Hypokalemia is attributed to ECF volume contraction which stimulates aldosterone and potassium secretion leading to increase urinary potassium loss.

2. Shift of Hydrogen Ions Intracellularly

Intracellular acidosis enhances bicarbonate reabsorption in the collecting duct. As the extracellular potassium concentration decreases, potassium ions move out of the cells. To maintain electroneutrality, hydrogen ions move into the intracellular space. Stimulation of the apical H^+/K^+ ATPase in the collecting duct leads to teleologically appropriate potassium ion reabsorption with corresponding hydrogen ion secretion. This leads to a net gain of bicarbonate, maintaining systemic alkalosis.

Stimulation of Renal Ammonia Genesis

Ammonium ions (NH_4^+) are produced in the proximal tubule from the metabolism of glutamine. During this process, alpha ketoglutarate is produced, the metabolism of which generates bicarbonate and is returned to the systemic circulation.

3. Impaired Chloride ion reabsorption in the distal Nephron

This results in an increase in luminal electronegativity, with subsequent enhancement of hydrogen ion secretion.

4. Reduction in Glomerular Filtration Rate (GFR)

This has been proven in animal studies. Hypokalemia by unknown mechanisms decreases GFR, which in turn decreases the filtered load of bicarbonate. In the presence of volume depletion, this impairs renal excretion of the excess bicarbonate

5. The Associated Chloride Deficiency

This leads to more severe forms of sustained metabolic alkalosis. Chloride depletion also causes extracellular fluid volume contraction resulting in reduction of glomerular filtration rate and HCO_3 filtration. This is combined with avid sodium and HCO_3 reabsorption and potassium secretion. The potassium depletion in turn stimulates tubular secretion of H^+ ions with increased excretion of titratable acid and ammonium in the urine. Chloride depletion also impairs secretion of HCO_3 into the distal nephron through Cl^-/HCO_3 exchanger. Administration of chloride corrects the alkalosis.

6. Alkali Administration

Administration of sodium bicarbonate in amounts that exceed the capacity of the kidneys to excrete the excess bicarbonate may cause metabolic alkalosis. This capacity is reduced when a reduction in filtered bicarbonate occurs, as observed in renal failure. When body stores of chloride and potassium are reduced, exogenous alkali administration leads to metabolic alkalosis. This can occur even if the kidney functions are normal.

7. Aluminum Hydroxide and Sodium Polystyrene Sulfonate (Kayexalate) Administration

Administration of aluminum hydroxide when combined with potassium exchange resin, sodium polystyrene sulfonate (kayexalate) leads to metabolic alkalosis. The gastric acid (H^+ ions) is neutralized by the aluminum hydroxide. When neutralized gastric contents reaches the distal duodenum, H^+ is not available for neutralizing the alkaline GI secretions there. The aluminum binds to the resin in exchange of sodium. Thus complete reabsorption of sodium and bicarbonate occurs in the gut.

Congenital Chloride Diarrhea or Villous adenoma of the Colon:

These are rare gastrointestinal causes of chloride sensitive metabolic alkalosis characterized by enormous chloride loss from the gut. Continuous use of large doses of chloride may be essential to correct the metabolic alkalosis.

Diuretics

Diuretics act in the various segments of the nephron mainly by blocking reabsorption of Na^+ and Cl^-. Loop diuretics act in the TAL and inhibit the sodium potassium 2 chloride (NaKCC2) transport system. Thiazides block the Na^+Cl^- cotransport system in the distal nephron. Metalazone also acts like thiazides on the distal tubule. Because of the presence of Na in the distal tubule, exchange of K^+ for Na^+ occurs under the influence of aldosterone. Na and H^+ ions are also exchanged in this segment. So in long-term diuretic use, Cl^-, K^+ and H^+ are lost in the urine leading to metabolic alkalosis and hypokalemia. The mild metabolic alkalosis is maintained by ECF volume contraction and further K^+ depletion due to secondary hyperaldosteronism. When this is combined with near normal total body bicarbonate content, the serum HCO_3 concentration increases. Restoration of the ECF volume deficit with isotonic saline will correct metabolic alkalosis.

Gastrocystoplasty

In gastrocystoplasty, a part of the stomach is used to augment bladder capacity. Since the augumented bladder wall now respond to gastrin, chloride is secreted into the bladder and excreted in urine. Thus metabolic alkalosis is sustained. Such patients require long term chloride supplementation.

Posthypercapnia

Chronic respiratory acidosis is associated with a compensatory increase in H^+ ion secretion and therefore in renal HCO_3 reabsorption. This represents an appropriate response, since the rise in plasma HCO_3^- concentration returns the extracellular pH towards normal. Treatment with mechanical ventilation in this disorder can lead to a rapid reduction in $PaCO_2$. The plasma HCO_3 however remains elevated resulting in metabolic alkalosis. This is due to memory effect.

Memory effect: Hypercapnia induced stimulation of HCO_3^- will persist even after the $PaCO_2$ has been returned to normal, mechanism is not clear.

Memory effect: The hypercapnia induced stimulation of HCO_3^- will persists even after the $PaCO_2$ has been returned to normal, mechanism is not clear.

Rapid fall in $PaCO_2$ and increase in cerebral pH can produce serious neurological abnormality and death. Hence chronic hypercarbia should be reduced slowly.

Treatment consists of cautious saline administration to correct hypovolumia, correction of hypokalemia if present and the use of a carbonic anhydrase inhibitor, e.g. acetazolamide.

Case History 3

A 60-year-old chronic smoker is admitted with a one week history of fever, cough and drowsiness.

He is centrally cyanosed with an oxygen saturation of 65%. Chest X-ray shows over inflation and bronchiectatic cavities in both mid zones. He is administered oxygen and antibiotics and the SPO_2 rises to 92%. ABG results are pH

Interpretation of ABGs

pH	7.29
PCO_2	72
PO_2	58
HCO_3	32

What is the Acid-Base Disorder?

Step 1: pH 7.29, hence acidosis

Step 2: PCO_2 is raised suggesting respiratory acidosis

Step 3: PaO_2 is low indicating hypoxia

Step 4: Find out the expected bicarbonate for increase in PCO_2. Here expected bicarbonate = PCO_2 = 4 mmol/L rise for 10 mm Hg, rise in PCO_2 = 24 + 12.8 = 36.8

Step 5: Compare the obtained bicarbonate with expected bicarbonate. The obtained bicarbonate = 32 which is less than the expected bicarbonate 36.8 suggesting coexisting metabolic alkalosis.

Despite additional oxygen supplementation the patient appears increasingly breathless. He is started on noninvasive ventilation by face mask. On an inspired oxygen concentration of 35% the SPO_2 picks up to 97%. The patient tolerates the mask, his respiratory rate decreases and he appears settled.

ABG values on the next day:

The ABG values on the next day are as follows:

pH	7.48
$PaCO_2$	48 mm Hg
PO_2	70 mm Hg
HCO_3	35 mEq/L

Step 1: pH 7.48, hence alkalosis

Step 2: $PaCO_2$ is 48, since $PaCO_2$ and HCO_3 is increased with alkaline pH, primary change is metabolic.

Step 3: PaO_2 is 70 and is in normal range

> **Step 4:** Bicarbonate is 35 indicating metabolic alkalosis
> **Step 5:** Compare the obtained $PaCO_2$ with expected $PaCO_2$
> The expected $PaCO_2$ is $40 + (8 \times .7) = 45.6$ mm Hg
> The final diagnosis is metabolic alkalosis with respiratory acidosis.

Patient who was admitted with respiratory alkalosis and metabolic acidosis, after correction of respiratory acidosis with ventilator support, developed metabolic alkalosis.

Comment

There is a gratifying decrease in carbon dioxide tension and improvement in oxygenation. The HCO_3 has increased in spite of the fall in $PaCO_2$ leading to a metabolic alkalosis. This could be due to

- Hypochloremia and hypokalemia from diuresis
- Posthypercapnic metabolic alkalosis

The patient was not on diuretic and there was no cardiac failure or edema. The probable diagnosis here is *Posthypercapnic metabolic alkalosis*.

The patient was treated with acetazolamide 125 mg twice daily. Patient was taken off noninvasive ventilation the next day. He remained mildly hypercapnic and hypoxic but was less dyspneic, afebrile and the pH decreased to 7.33. Kidney will take 2–3 days to decrease bicarbonate reabsorption.

METABOLIC ALKALOSIS AND NORMAL OR EXPANDED ECF VOLUME

Metabolic alkalosis with normal or expanded ECF volume can have high blood pressure. If the fluid accumulation is not severe, edema may not be present. Patients with normal ECF volume or ECF volume contraction will have normal or low blood pressure. Common causes are the use of diuretics like thiazides, frusemide, rare causes are Bartter syndrome and Gitelman syndrome. In such situation serum K^+ measurement will give clue to the diagnosis.

Case History 4

A two-year-old child weighing 8 kg is admitted with feeble cry, polyuria, polydipsia, vomiting, constipation, salt craving, tendency for volume depletion, failure to thrive, and linear growth retardation. Child was clinically euvolemic and blood pressure normal for age. Investigations are as follows.

Parameters in blood/serum	Values
Blood urea	20 mg%
Creatinine	0.5 mg%
Na	122 mmol/L
K	3 mmol/L
Chloride	96 mmol/L
Bicarbonate	28 mmol/L
Mg	1.5 mEq/L

Child has hyponatremia, hypokalemia, hypochloremia, and raised-bicarbonate. ABG values are shown below

pH	7.40
PCO$_2$	46 mm Hg
HCO$_3$	28 mmol/L
PaO$_2$	70 mm Hg

Steps

1. Interpret the pH 7.40, normal range 7.35–7.45. Normal pH and elevated bicarbonate indicate a mixed acid-base disorder.
2. Correlate with HCO$_3$. Bicarbonate is above the normal range 22–24 mmol/L, indicates retention of bicarbonate, hence metabolic alkalosis.
3. What is his PaCO$_2$? 46 mm Hg (above normal 40 mm Hg). In this child plasma HCO$_3$ is 28 mmol/L. Expected increase in PaCO$_2$ is (28 – 24) × 0.7 = 2.8. So the expected PaCO$_2$ is 40 + 2.8 = 42.8 mm Obtained PaCO$_2$ is 46 mm, suggesting a coexistent respiratory acidosis. Patient has normal blood pressure, euvolumia metabolic alkalosis, and respiratory acidosis.
4. Estimation of loss of potassium in urine will give a clue to diagnosis. Urinary loss is less than 10 mmol/L suggest non-renal causes

In the child (case history 4), find out urinary potassium loss.

Urine electrolytes are as follows

Electrolytes in urine	mmol/L
Na	35
K	20 mEq
Chloride	25
Calcium	40 mg in 24 hours (normal 4 mg/kg)

Child has metabolic alkalosis, respiratory acidosis, hyponatremia, hypokalemia, hypochloremia with urinary loss of Na, K and chloride.

There is no history of diuretic intake or other known cause for hypokalemia. Bartter's syndrome and Gitelman's syndrome are the differential diagnosis.

To differentiate Bartter from Gittelman's syndrome.

Urinary calcium and plasma Mg is done.

Child has normal Mg and is hypercalciuric, and the final diagnosis is Bartter's syndrome.

Approach to metabolic alkalosis in patients with normal/low blood pressure and ECF volume based on urine potassium loss is shown in Figure 19.4. Bartter's syndrome and Gitelman's syndrome are discussed in chapter on hypokalemia.

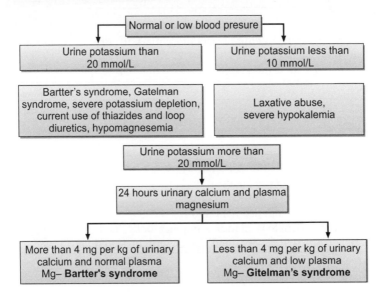

Fig. 19.4: Causes in patients with normal or low BP and ECF volume based on urine potassium loss

Case History 5

A 20-year-old male presented to the emergency ward with severe headache. On physical examination, he was euvolemic. The blood pressure in the 4 limbs were RUL 160/120, LUL 150/110, RLL 180/114 and LLL 180/116. There was no papilledema or renal bruit.

Parameters in blood/serum	Values
Blood urea	30 mg%
Creatinine	0.9 mg%
Na	140 mmol /L
K	2.5 mmol/L
Chloride	86 mmol/L
Bicarbonate	28 mmol/L

Patient is euvolumic. The laboratory parameters showed normal GFR, with hypokalemia, hypochloremia, and raised bicarbonate.

Step 1: Check urine potassium

Urine electrolytes are as follows

Electrolytes in urine	Mmol/L
Na	20
K	30
Chloride	60

Patient has hypokalemia, hypochloremia with urinary potassium and chloride loss.

ABG values are shown below

pH	7.46
PCO_2	43 mm Hg
HCO_3	28 mmol/L
PaO_2	98 mm Hg

Stepwise Approach to ABG Analysis

Step 1: pH 7.46 hence alkalosis

Step 2: $PaCO_2$ 43 is raised

Step 3: PaO_2 98 is in normal range

Step 4: Bicarbonate is 28 indicating metabolic alkalosis

Step 5: Compare the obtained $PaCO_2$ with expected $PaCO_2$.

The expected $PaCO_2$ is 28 + 15 = 43. Here the obtained $PaCO_2$ and the expected $PaCO_2$ are identical = 43 mm Hg suggesting simple metabolic alkalosis.

Patient has Hypertension, metabolic alkalosis with hypokalemia, hypochloremia, urinary loss of Na, K, and chloride.

Approach to metabolic alkalosis in patients with normal/expanded ECF volume is shown in Figure 19.5.

Step 4: To check renin and aldosterone levels. Patient had low renin and high aldosterone and diagnosis is primary hyperaldosteronism Conn's syndrome.

Diagnosis was confirmed by CT scan which showed adrenal adenoma. Treatment consists of spironolactone for correction of hypertension, hypokalemia and surgical resection of adenoma.

SALINE RESISTANT METABOLIC ALKALOSIS (FIG. 19.5)

The pathogenesis of saline resistant metabolic alkalosis is centered round mineralocorticoid excess. This is often associated with extracellular volume expansion, hypertension, hypokalemia, urinary chloride > 15 mmol/L, hypermineralocorticoidism and non-responsiveness to chloride administration. The mineralocorticoid excess or abnormalities in the renal tubular transport are the main factors in the pathogenesis. The three important transport systems in the nephron are

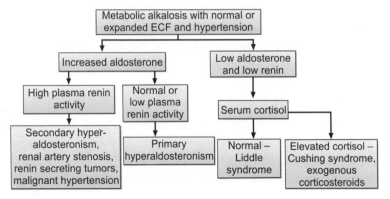

Fig. 19.5: Causes in patients with expanded ECF volume, hypertension based on aldosterone

NaKCC2 cotransporter in the TAL, Na^+-Cl^- cotransport in the distal tubule and aldostorone regulated Na, K counter transport in the distal tubule.

Mineralocorticoid excess causes increase in net acid excretion and when this is combined with K^+ deficiency results in sustained metabolic alkalosis. Na^+ retention causes ECF volume expansion and hypertension. ECF volume expansion increases GFR and tubular acidification. The aldosterone effect and consequent K^+ secretion also increases tubular acidification. The K^+ loss causes polyuria due to inability to concentrate the urine.

Hyperaldosteronism

Aldosterone and other mineralocorticoids increase H^+ ATPase activity and cause excretion of H^+ ions and alkalosis. By acting on epithelial Na^+ channels in the collecting duct, they cause sodium retention, potassium wasting and hypertension. Alkalosis is mild ($HCO_3 \sim 30$ mml/L) but hypokalemia is severe (often < 3 mmol/L). Isolated mineralocorticoid excess or those associated with excess of other adrenocortical hormones as shown in Figure 19.5 can be responsible.

Administration of mineralocorticoids including fludrocortisone or excess endogenous production, increases net acid excretion and result in metabolic alkalosis. Associated K^+ deficiency may worsen the same. Hyperaldosteronism may be due to primary overproduction (Conn's syndrome) or secondary to renin secretion.

Hyper-reninemic States

Renal artery stenosis either unilateral or bilateral, accelerated hypertension, renin secreting tumors or estrogen therapy are associated with high levels of renin which stimulate the reninangiotensin aldosterone axis and increase aldosterone levels.

Enzyme Deficiencies

11 β hydroxysteroid dehydrogenase deficiency is a rare familial syndrome of apparent mineralocorticoid excess. It is caused by mutation of the gene leading to inactivation of the enzyme 11 β hydroxysteroid dehydrogenase. This enzyme normally minimizes cortisol binding to the receptor which converts cortisol to cortisone. When this enzyme is inactivated, cortisol activates the receptor causing sodium reabsorption and K^+ secretion leading to Cl^- resistant metabolic alkalosis with hypertension and low aldostorone levels.

Carbenoxolene and licorice also inhibit the activity of 11 β hydrosteroid dehydrogenase.

17 α Hydroxylase Deficiency

17-hydroxylase (17-OH) deficiency syndrome is a rare genetic disorder of steroid biosynthesis that causes decreased production of glucocorticoids and sex steroids and increased synthesis of mineralocorticoid precursors. Mineralocorticoid excess produces varying degrees of metabolic alkalosis, hypertension and hypokalemia. Patients usually present with delayed puberty, absent secondary sexual characteristics, or primary amenorrhea.

Management of Metabolic Alkalosis

This is primarily based on the underlying etiology and the patient's volume status. If vomiting is the cause administer antiemetics. In patients on continuous gastric suction H_2-blockers/proton-pump inhibitors are indicated. In patients, on thiazide or loop diuretics, the dose can be reduced or the drug can be stopped. If diuretics are essential potassium-sparing diuretics or acetazolamide may be used.

CHLORIDE-RESPONSIVE ALKALOSIS

Patients with volume depletion can be managed with an intravenous infusion of isotonic sodium chloride solution.

Since, this is usually associated with hypokalemia, potassium chloride should also be added to correct the hypokalemia. In edematous states [e.g. congestive heart failure (CHF)], use potassium chloride instead of sodium chloride to *avoid volume overload.* If diuresis is needed, a carbonic anhydrase inhibitor (e.g. acetazolamide) or a potassium-sparing diuretic (e.g. spironolactone, amiloride, triamterene) can be used.

Chloride-Resistant Metabolic Alkalosis

Management is based on the specific cause.

Primary hyperaldosteronism—Medical treatment consists **of** Aldosterone antagonist spironolactone or with other potassium-sparing diuretics (e.g., amiloride, triamterene). If the cause of primary hyperaldosteronism is an adrenal adenoma or carcinoma, surgical removal of the tumor is indicated. **In glucocorticoid-remediable hyperaldosteronism,** Dexamethasone can be given.

In **Cushing syndrome** potassium-sparing diuretics offers temporary relief. *Definitive* therapy is transsphenoidal microresection of adrenocorticotropic hormone (ACTH)—producing pituitary adenomas and adrenalectomy for adrenal tumors. In **syndrome of apparent mineralocorticoid excess** potassium-sparing diuretics along with dexamethasone may be used to suppress cortisol production by inhibiting ACTH. Unlike cortisol and some synthetic glucocorticoids, **dexamethasone does not activate the mineralocorticoid receptor.**

In **Bartter's syndrome and Gitelman's syndrome management is** partially with potassium supplementation, potassium-sparing diuretics, non-steroidal anti-inflammatory drugs, or ACE inhibitors. Potassium-sparing diuretics if used should be amiloride or triamterene, *but not spironolactone.* Both amiloride and triamterene inhibit the apical sodium ion channel in the collecting duct. Spironolactone, which is a mineralocorticoid receptor antagonist that works upstream of the defective sodium ion channel, does not correct the alkalosis or the hypertension.

Specialized Therapies in All Types of Metabolic Alkalosis Hydrochloric Acid-Indications

When pH > 7.55 and/or when sodium or potassium chloride cannot be administered because of volume overload or advanced renal failure. Rapid correction of severe metabolic alkalosis is warranted (e.g. cardiac arrhythmias, hepatic encephalopathy, digoxin cardiotoxicity).

Ammonium Chloride

Ammonium chloride is administered to correct severe metabolic alkalosis related to chloride deficiency. NH_4Cl is converted to ammonia and HCl by the liver. By releasing HCl, NH_4Cl may help to correct metabolic alkalosis. This agent is available as 500 mg tablets and a 26.75% parenteral formulation for intravenous use. The parenteral formulation contains 5 mEq/mL (267.5 mg/mL).

Indication for Dialysis

In advanced renal failure, who usually have volume overload and are resistant to acetazolamide, acetate-free biofiltration (buffer-free dialysate), in which bicarbonate is not present in the dialysate is used. But is infused separately as needed. Peritoneal dialysis can be performed using isotonic sodium chloride solution as the dialysate.

KEY POINTS

- Metabolic alkalosis is an associated abnormality and not a primary disorder.
- Common cause is volume contraction and treatment is saline infusion.
- Urine chloride and urine potassium values are clues to the correct diagnosis.

- Metabolic alkalosis may be associated with ECF volume contraction, normal ECF or with ECF volume expansion.
- Estimation of urinary loss of potassium will give a clue to the diagnosis of primary disorder.
- In patients of hypertension, estimation of PRA and aldosterone will add to the diagnosis.
- Management of metabolic alkalosis in general depends on volume status, underlying etiology and clinical symptoms.

Case Histories

A Vimala

CASE HISTORY 1

A 50-year-old lady was admitted with complaints of sudden onset of difficulty in breathing. Patient gives history of loose watery stools for two days prior to admission. Significant past history includes type 2 DM. On examination pulse was not felt, BP was not recordable. She was acidotic. Systemic examination was unremarkable. Her weight was 50 kg.

Parameters	On Admission
Urine	
Protein	+ +
Acetone	+
Hb, TC	13.9, 14200 (N9 3 L)
FBS	445 mg/DL
Blood urea	55 mg/dL
S. Creatinine	0.8 mg/dL
S. Na	140 mmol/L
S. K	3 mmol/L
S. Cl	115 mmol/L
S. Alb	3.6 g/dL

How do you manage? Patient had uncontrolled hyperglycemia probably with underlying infection as suggested by neutrophilic leukocytosis. She has normal creatinine with disproportionate elevation of urea. Sodium when corrected for hyperglycemia is 145 mmol/L and potassium is low. This indicates severe degree of dehydration. Probable cause for hypovolemia in this patient is osmotic diuresis due to hyperglycemia, diarrheal loss and decreased fluid intake.

ABG parameters	On the day of admission
pH	6.982
PCO_2	12.8
PO_2	176.9 (FiO_2 40%)
BE	–26.8
BE ecf	–28.5
HCO_3	2.9 mmol/L
O_2 sat	97.8

Analysis of ABG Report

Steps

1. pH is 6.982 is very low, hence has acidosis.
2. HCO_3 2.9 mmol/L is very low, has metabolic acidosis.
3. Expected PCO_2 is 18 (for every mmol decrease in HCO_3, PCO_2 decreases by 1 mm). Here, the PCO_2 is 12.8 lower, than the expected value suggesting coexistent respiratory alkalosis.
4. Calculate the Anion gap, AG = 140 – (115 + 2.9) = 22, AG is increased, hence anion gap metabolic acidosis (AGMA).
5. Compare Δ AG and Δ HCO_3,
   Δ AG = observed AG - normal AG = 22 – 12 = 10,
   Δ HCO_3 = normal HCO_3 - patient's HCO_3 = 24 – 3 = 21
   Reduction in HCO_3 is due to additon of H^+ ions.
   Δ HCO_3 is much more than Δ AG, indicates there are two processes, the addition of inorganic acid containing chloride which is a measured anion hence will not change AG, and also the addition of organic acid anion which

is not measured and has changed AG. Diagnosis-hybrid metabolic acidosis – combination of HCMA with AGMA.

6. Interpret PaO_2, always in relation to FiO_2.

Patient on FiO_2 0.40, PaO_2/FiO_2 177/0.4 = 442 – normal.

Treatment Given

Patient was dehydrated and in shock, hence the intravascular volume was expanded with normal saline 1 liter in the first hour and 500 mL/h till blood pressure normalized. Since the pH was less than 7.1 sodium bicarbonate was infused. Dose of HCO_3 required was calculated as follows

Target pH is 7.1. pH of 7.1 corresponds to H^+ ion concentration of 80 nmol/L. According to Handerson's equation $H^+ = 24 \times PCO_2/HCO_3^-$ Assuming that PCO_2 has not changed, the HCO_3^- required to lower the H^+ ions to 80, 24 × 12.8 /80 = 3.84 HCO_3^- deficit = 3.84 – 2.9 = 1 mmol/L.

Since the patient is severely acidotic, the bicarbonate space that has to be corrected is 100% of body weight.

Total HCO_3^- deficit = 50 × 1 = 50 mmole/L.

Volume of 7.5% HCO_3^- required = 50/0.9 = 55 mL

This was infused rapidly.

Hyperglycemia was controlled with insulin infusion.

Hypokalemia was corrected with potassium citrate solution.

CASE HISTORY 2

A young woman presented with a history of watery diarrhea two days after a railway journey. She is febrile, tachycardic, has dry mouth and cold extremities. Her blood pressure was 90/60 mm Hg.

What is the ABG Diagnosis on Clinical Grounds?

Since patient is hypotensive, there may be reduced tissue perfusion, poor tissue oxygenation and anaerobic metabolism resulting in lactic acidosis. Loss of bicarbonate rich intestinal fluid in diarrhea can result in non-AG metabolic acidosis. Patient may also have respiratory alkalosis due to infection.

Investigations

Blood urea	40 mg/dL
S. creatinine	1.4 mg/dL
S. Na	135 mmol/L
S. K	2.8 mmol/L
S. Cl	108 mmol/L
S. HCO_3	18 mmol/L
Anion gap	9 mmol/L
Albumin	2.5 g/dL
Corrected AG	$9 + 2 \times (4.5 - 2.5) = 13$

Patient has normal creatinine, reduced potassium with corrected AG of 13.

ABG Analysis

pH	7.31
PCO_2	35 mm Hg
PO_2	95 on room air
HCO_3	16 mmol/L
O_2 sat	95%

Analysis of ABG Report

Steps
1. pH 7.31 is low, hence acidosis.
2. HCO_3 16 mmol/L is low, indicates metabolic acidosis.
3. Expected PCO_2 is 32 (for every mmol decrease in HCO_3, PCO_2 decreases by 1 mm). Here the PCO_2 is 35, higher than the expected value suggesting coexistent respiratory acidosis.
4. Calculate the anion gap. AG = 135 – (108 + 18) = 9. corrected AG is 13.

This indicates non-anion gap metabolic acidosis. Hypokalemia due to diarrhea has produced respiratory muscle fatigue and mild respiratory acidosis.

CASE HISTORY 3

An insulin dependent diabetic patient stopped taking insulin for 2 days and presented to casualty with vomiting and breathlessness. He complaints of severe thirst. On examination his BP was 100/70 mm Hg, pulse rate 110/min, regular and had acidotic breathing. Systemic examination was otherwise unremarkable.

Clinical diagnosis: Patient has diabetic ketoacidosis.

Investigations

Blood sugar	300 mg/dL
S. Creatinine	1.4 mg/dL
S. Na	135 mmol/L
S. K	5 mmol/L
S. Cl	100 mmol/L
S. HCO$_3$	12 mmol/L
Anion gap	23 mmol/L
S. Albumin	3.5 g/dl
Corrected AG	23 + 2 × (4.5 − 3.5) = 25
Urine ketones	positive

ABG Analysis

pH	7.25
PCO$_2$	27 mm Hg
PO$_2$	81 on room air
HCO$_3$	12 mmol/L
O$_2$ sat	95%

Interpretation of ABG

Steps

1. pH 7.25 is low, hence acidosis.
2. HCO$_3$ is 12 mmol/L is low and has metabolic acidosis.

3. Expected PCO_2 is 27 mm Hg and is same as observed PCO_2 and hence has simple metabolic acidosis.
4. Calculate the anion gap, AG = 135 – (100 + 12) = 23 and corrected AG is 23 + 2 = 25.
5. Compare Δ AG and delta HCO_3,
   Δ AG = observed AG – normal AG = 25 – 12 =13.
   Δ HCO_3 = normal HCO_3 – patient's HCO_3 = 24 – 12 = 12,
   Δ HCO_3 is almost equal to Δ AG. This is suggestive of AGMA. The AG is increased because of the accumulation of organic acid probably ketoacid which is unmeasured.
6. Interpret PaO_2 always in relation to FiO_2 patient is on room air and PaO_2 is 81 mm Hg.
   PaO_2/FiO_2 ratio is 81/0.21 = 400, normal.

Diagnosis is *anion gap metabolic acidosis-diabetic ketoacidosis. She was managed with insulin and IV fluids.*

CASE HISTORY 4

A 65-year-old woman who has been diabetic and hypertensive for 5 years on oral hypoglycemic agents and indapamide developed cellulitis of the foot following injury 15 days prior to admission. She was admitted with complaints of muscle weakness. On examination patient was hypovolemic BP 110/70 mm Hg, hypotonia with grade 4 muscle power in all four limbs.

Investigations

Blood sugar	360 mg/dL
S. Creatinine	1.2 mg/dL
S. Na	132 mmol/L
S. K	2.6 mmol/L
S. Cl	82 mmol/L
S. HCO_3	18 mmol/L
Anion gap	32
S. Albumin	4.5 g /dL
Corrected AG	32

ABG Analysis

pH	7.41
PCO_2	32 mm Hg
PO_2	71 on room air
HCO_3	20 mmol/L
O_2 sat	95%

Interpret These Values

Steps

1. pH 7.41, normal range—can be normal or a mixed acid-base disorder towards alkalosis.
2. PCO_2 is 32 mm Hg indicating respiratory alkalosis.
3. HCO_3 20 mmol/L is low. Expected HCO_3 for PCO_2 of 32 is 23.4. Observed HCO_3 is low indicating coexistant metabolic acidosis.
4. Calculate the anion gap, AG = 132 – (82 + 18) = 32.
5. Compare Δ AG and Δ HCO_3,
   Δ AG = observed AG - normal AG = 32 – 12 = 20,
   Δ HCO_3 = normal HCO_3 - patient's HCO_3 = 24 – 18 = 6
   Δ HCO_3 is less than Δ AG, indicating the addition of alkali, pre-existing metabolic alkalosis or a chronic compensated respiratory acidosis.
6. Interpret PaO_2, always in relation to FiO_2, patient on room air 81 mm Hg PaO_2/FiO_2 71/0.21 = 355, normal.

In this patient, the Indapamide (diuretic antihypertensive agent) must be the cause for the metabolic alkalosis and low potassium. She has a high anion gap metabolic acidosis due DKA and mild respiratory alkalosis.

CASE HISTORY 5

A 75-year-old man with a longstanding history of heavy smoking is brought to hospital in a febrile and confused state. He rapidly becomes drowsy. SPO_2 is 80%. Clinical assessment indicates the patient is likely to have a chronic respiratory acidosis. He is hypoxic, so there is a possibility of lactic acidosis in addition.

Investigations

Blood sugar	120 mg/dL
S. Creatinine	1 mg//dL
S. Na	134 mmol/L
S. K	5 mmol/L
S. Cl	82 mmol/L
S. HCO_3	29 mmol/L

ABG Analysis

PH	7.21
PCO_2	70 mm hg
pO_2	55 on room air
HCO_3	26 mmoles/L
O_2 sat	80%

Interpret These Values

Step 1: pH 7.21 is low, hence acidosis.

Step 2: HCO_3 26 mmol/L, is high, look at PCO_2.

Step 3: PCO_2 is 70, suggesting accumulation of CO_2 — respiratory acidosis.

Step 4: Interpret PaO_2, always in relation to FiO_2, patient on room air 55 mm Hg.

PaO_2/FiO_2 55/0.21 = 275, abnormal.

Step 5: Expected HCO_3^- the renal compensation for a chronic rise in PCO_2 of 30 (70 – 40) should be 3.5 × 3 = 10.5, so the HCO_3 should have been 24 + 10.5 = 34.5 mmol/L. Here the bicarbonate is only 26 mmol/L, There is therefore a metabolic acidosis also.

Step 6: Anion gap 134 – (82 + 29) = 23.

The Δ ratio need not be calculated (we already know there is a respiratory acidosis) and the bicarbonate is increased above the normal of 24, not decreased.

The patient has chronic respiratory acidosis due to chronic obstructive lung disease and metabolic acidosis due to possible lactic acid accumulation in hypoxia.

CASE HISTORY 6

A 50-year-old man was admitted with a 3-day history of abdominal pain and vomiting. The patient was pale and tachypneic, blood pressure was not recordable and the abdomen was rigid. He was resuscitated with IV fluids and taken up for emergency laparotomy which revealed infected ascitic fluid and a perforated duodenal ulcer.

Diagnosis

Shock with peritonitis due to a duodenal perforation.

Investigations

WBC	14500/mm^3
Hb	14 g
Blood sugar	102 mg/dL
Creatinine	0.8 mg/dL
Na	129 mmol/L
K	4.4 mmol/L
Cl	84 mmol/L
HCO$_3$	15 mmol/L
Case histories	257

ABG Analysis

pH	7.21
PCO$_2$	39 mm Hg
PO$_2$	85% on room air
HCO$_3$	14.6 mmol/L
O$_2$sat	80%

Interpret These Values

Step 1: pH 7.21 is low, hence acidosis.

Step 2: HCO_3 15 mmol/L is low, metabolic acidosis.

Step 3: Expected PCO_2 is 27 to 31 (Winter's formula: PCO_2 should be $14.6 \times 1.5 + 8 \pm 2 = 27$ to 31, obtained PCO_2 is 39 more than expected indicating coexistent respiratory acidosis.

Step 4: Calculate the anion gap, $AG = 124 - (84 + 15) = 25$.

Step 5: Compare ΔAG and ΔHCO_3,

ΔAG = observed AG - normal AG = $25 - 12 = 13$,

ΔHCO_3 = normal HCO_3 - patient's $HCO_3 = 24 - 14.6 = 9.4$.

ΔHCO_3 is less than ΔAG, indicating the addition of alkali, a pre-existing metabolic alkalosis or a chronic compensated respiratory acidosis.

Step 6: Interpret PaO_2 always in relation to FiO_2, patient on room air 81 mm Hg.

PaO_2/FiO_2 85/0.21 = 425, normal.

The patient has a high anion gap metabolic acidosis from septic shock and a respiratory acidosis due to diaphragmatic splinting from peritonitis. A serum lactate level would help to confirm lactic acidosis.

CASE HISTORY 7

A 45-year-old male patient diagnosed to have post-infective glomerulonephritis and alcoholic liver disease was admitted with spontaneous bacterial peritonitis. O/E generalized edema, BP-130/90 mm Hg.

On admission investigations are as follows.

Hb	5.8 g%
TC	12500/cmm
D C	N90, L10
S. Na	131 mmol/L
S. K+	2.8 mmol/L

Contd...

Contd...

Cl⁻	86 mmol/L
S. K⁺	5.9 mmol/L
Creatinine	3.3 mg%
Albumin	2 g%

Impression

A/C kidney injury in a patient with low ECF volume, due to third space loss and expected abnormalities are anion gap metabolic acidosis because of kidney and liver disease. Sepsis can produce lactic acidosis. Diuretics and vomiting can induce metabolic alkalosis, and hepatic failure also can produce respiratory alkalosis.

ABG Analysis on Admission

PH	7.596
PCO₂	34.1
PO₂	46.7 (on room air)
BE	9.9
HCO₃	32.5
O₂sat	90.5

Interpret These Values

Step 1: pH 7.596, high hence alkalosis.

Step 2: HCO_3 32.5 mmol/L, is high, metabolic alkalosis.

Step 3: Expected PCO_2 is 46 (PCO_2 should be 40 + (32.5 – 24) × 0.7, obtained PCO_2 is 34. 1 less than expected indicating coexistent respiratory alkalosis.

Step 4: Calculate the anion gap, AG = 131– (86 + 32.5) = 12.5, corrected AG = 12.5 + 2 × 2.5 = 17.5.

Step 5: Interpret PaO_2 always in relation to FiO_2, patient on room air 46.7 mm Hg.

PaO_2/FiO_2 46.7/0.21 = 240, indicates acute lung injury.

This patient has metabolic alkalosis, metabolic acidosis as evidenced by increase in AG and respiratory alkalosis with hypoxia.

CASE HISTORY 8

A 60-year-old lady is admitted with complaints of anorexia and diarrhea. Significant past illness included type II DM, hypertension, chronic osteomyelitis and recurrent urinary tract infection. O/E volume status—Dehydrated, BP 110/80 mm Hg, no evidence of active osteomyelitis.

Investigations (On Admission)

Urine-protein—2+, WBC—numerous, Hb—9.94%, TC—17600, DC—Na_1 L_6EO_3.

Parameter	On Admission	After 48 hours
RBS	410 mg	167 mg
Urea	218	199
Creatinine	4.3	4.2
Na	119	131
K^+	7.2	4.8
Cl^-	96	98
AG	13	19
Albumin	2.5 g	3 g
Corrected AG	16	22
pH	7.193	7.267
pCO_2	25.6	31.4
HCO_{3-}	9.6	14
PaO_2	109 mm Hg	114.7
O_2sat	93%	95%

Interpretation

Urinalysis shows pyuria with culture positive for *E. coli*. Hemogram showing anemia and polymorphonuclear leukocytosis

Biochemical Investigations

Moderate kidney failure and uncontrolled hyperglycemia.

Electrolytes

Low sodium- Hyperglycemia can dilute Na^+ and correction factor is for every 100 mg above normal value of 100 mg of glucose, sodium will decrease by 1.6. So, expected Na^+ in this patient due to hyperglycemia is 140 – (3 × 1.6) = 135. Patient's Na^+ is 119, suggesting severe hyponatremia.

ABG Analysis

Step 1: PH-7.193 indicates acidosis.
Step 2: Correlate it with bicarbonate (HCO_3 9.6)- bicarbonate is low indicates metabolic acidosis.
Step 3: Expected decrease in PCO_2 for HCO_3 of 9.6 is 9 × 1.5 + 8 ± 2.

So the expected PCO_2, 19 to 23. The observed PCO_2 is 25.6 more than expected suggesting respiratory acidosis.
Step 4: Compare with Δ anion gap with Δ HCO_3^-.

HCO_3 = (normal HCO_3^- – observed HCO_3
= (24 – 9.6) = 14.4.
Anion gap = Na^+ – (Cl^- + HCO_3) = 119 – (96 + 9.6) = 13.4

Corrected anion gap = (observed anion gap) + (4.5 – 2.5) × 2 = 17.4

Indicating anion gap metabolic acidosis (AGMA)
Δ AG = (Observed AG - Normal AG) = 18 – 12 = 6
Δ HCO_3 of 14.4 > Δ AG 6 **Indicating hybrid metabolic acidosis** (The combination of normal hyperchloremic metabolic acidosis with anion gap metabolic acidosis).

In this patient, AGMA is due to DKA and normal AG acidosis is due to diarrhea. Patient was managed with insulin infusion, normal saline infusion and antibiotics.

Since GFR was > 25 mL/min and K^+ was high in association with HCMA, possibility is type IV renal tubular acidosis (RTA) (due to acute interstitial nephritis). Patient was also started on 100 µg of fludrocortisone.

48 hours after admission hyperglycemia was controlled. and pH increased to 7.26.

Bottom Line

- Whenever there is hybrid metabolic acidosis exclude comorbid conditions like diarrhea, type IV RTA, etc.
- Severe hyperkalemia with moderate decrease in GFR suggest type IV RTA and fludrocortisone may be beneficial.
- Sodium bicarbonate infusionis indicated only when pH is less than 7 in DKA.

Bibliography

1. Feehally J, et al (Eds). Comprehensive Clinical Nephrology, 4th edition. Mosby, London, 2010.
2. Halperin M, Goldstein MC. Fluid, Electrolyte and Acid-base Physiology—Problem Based Approach, 3rd edition. Philadelphia: WB Saunders Company, 1999.
3. Harrison's Principles of Internal Medicine, 18th edition.
4. Schrier RW, Kluwer W (Eds). Renal and Electrolyte Disorders, 7th edition. Philadelphia: Lippincott Williams and Wilkins, 2010.

Index

Page numbers followed by *f* refer to figure and *t* refer to table